MW00965289

GOD'S REMEDY

GOD'S REMEDY

How to Really Recover from Fibromyalgia, Myofascial Pain Syndrome, Chronic Fatigue Syndrome, CFIDS, Gulf War Syndrome, Anxiety (Panic) Attacks, and Other Chronic Muscle Pain Conditions

The First Book ever with the Newest and latest Revolutionary Breakthrough
discovery showing you step by step how to Effectively Eliminate:
Constant Widespread Musculoskeletal Pain
Tender Points
Trigger Points and Anxiety (Panic) Attacks

While Minimizing:
Fatigue and Insomnia

BISHOP ROD GATTI

Forward by Keith N. Shenberger, M.D., FACR, FACP

Copyright © 2009 by Bishop Rod Gatti.

Library of Congress Control Number:		2009902816
ISBN:	Hardcover	978-1-4415-2246-7
	Softcover	978-1-4415-2245-0

All rights reserved. No part of this book may be reproduced or transmitted in any form or by any means, electronic or mechanical, including photocopying, recording, or by any information storage and retrieval system, without permission in writing from the copyright owner.

This book was printed in the United States of America.

To order additional copies of this book, contact:
Xlibris Corporation
1-888-795-4274
www.Xlibris.com
Orders@Xlibris.com
50592

CONTENTS

ILLUSTRATIONS

To my wife, Cathy, who has a special gift as a nurturing caregiver, my family who was there for me when I suddenly became ill, and to all of those who suffer from these painful conditions.

Fatigue, muscle pain and Anxiety (Panic) Attacks may be caused by illnesses other than Fibromyalgia, Myofascial Pain Syndrome, Chronic Fatigue Syndrome or Gulf War Syndrome, etc. Always consult with your physician before arriving at any conclusion concerning your medical condition for proper diagnosis and treatment. Also consult with your physician before starting any and all medication, herbal, diet and exercise regimens.

The information contained in this book is not intended to diagnose, treat, cure or prevent any illness or disease. Any and all applications of ideas, suggestions and/or procedures will be at the reader's own discretion.

FORWARD

This is a book about healing and attaining wholeness. Those who ignore the spiritual realm of life do so at their own risk. Any chronic illness, fully developed, causes physical, psychological and spiritual disturbances, and the healing process must address all three parameters of disease to be fully successful. Many people are cured but not healed.

We as physicians often address the physiological and anatomic abnormalities of a patient's malady, leaving the spiritual and psychological aspects to, hopefully, heal themselves. These deeper forms of healing are much more challenging to address, for they often require the active involvement of the patient. No longer a passive participant in the clinical process, the sufferer must find the resources within himself to attain true wholeness.

Here is where religious faith often plays an active part. Mr. Gatti approaches the common syndromes of fibromyalgia and related disorders with a comprehensive program of diet and exercise, along with a generous helping of scriptually-based advice. He documents here his own dramatic improvement using the power of prayer and the victory over fear available through an adamantine religious faith. He shares with readers the insights resulting from his healing journey.

In recent years, traditional medical science has begun to be more sensitive to spiritual aspects of the healing process. Some preliminary investigations into the nature of the juncture between medical treatment and religious faith have been performed. This area of therapeutics is very challenging to investigate in a conventional way. Scientific and religious ways of knowing are deeply different in nature, and cannot be reconciled.

Anyone with an even passing acquaintance with the Bible knows of the many healing stories found in both Testaments-some very dramatic, indeed miraculous. Perhaps the most important overarching theme of the Christian Scriptures is the healing of the broken relationship between God and man. The historical mission of Jesus Christ was to provide reconciliation in a relationship that had been fractured in the Garden of Eden.

We can never overestimate the power of faith in improving health and recovering from illness. The Letter to the Hebrews defines faith as "the assurance of things hoped for, the conviction of things not seen" (chapter 11, verse 1, NRSV). This aspect of human existence is inherently non-scientific for it is not based on knowledge, but rather on belief-nevertheless it has strong effects in the life of the faithful. This part of being human is addressed very revealingly by Paul in his Letter to the Ephesians. He writes: "I pray that . . . he may grant that you may be strengthened in your inner being with power through his Spirit, and that Christ may dwell in your hearts by faith . . . (and you may) know the love of Christ that surpasses knowledge . . ."(chapter 3, verses 16,17 and 19, NRSV). Indeed, the whole process of attaining faith is a gift from God.

Paul concludes this section of his letter with a doxology which speaks directly to the aims of this book when he writes "Now to him by the power at work within us is able to accomplish far more than all we can ask or imagine, to him be glory . . . to all generations forever and ever" (verses 20 and 21, NRSV).

Those who suffer from the intractable pain and unrelenting fatigue of fibromyalgia will find comfort and good advice in these pages. Here Rod Gatti provides a program of recovery to attain wholeness on all levels.

Keith N. Shenberger M.D., FACR, FACP
Rheumatologist, Williamsport, PA.

PREFACE

There are an estimated 26 million people suffering with Fibromyalgia Syndrome (FMS) and/or Myofascial Pain Syndrome in the United States (Starlanyl and Copeland, 1996) and over 192 million worldwide (Consensus Document, 1992). It is also estimated that 10-20 times more women than men suffer from these disabling syndromes. Women from age 20-50 seem to be the most affected (Eichner, 1990). With this many people suffering, it's easy to understand why there is an increased interest in determining what causes them and what can possibly cure them. At minimum, give long-lasting effective treatment.

As a once-diagnosed patient of FMS, MPS, CFS and Anxiety (Panic) Attacks, I know first hand the devastation they can bring to a person's life. They are ruthless, vicious and indiscriminating in their attack. It can debilitate you quickly or progress slowly over time, until you lose your normal level of functioning.

Until now, no one knew of a treatment or cure that could put into remission the musculoskeletal pain, virtually all fatigue, tender points and trigger points simultaneously. And these results were achieved without the use of medication(s). Currently, I need no further treatment for these syndromes. I have put FMS, MPS, CFS and AA, behind me the best I could and am moving on with my life as a victor, rather than a victim. The scars are there, but for the most part, they are healed over. Like the Bible says in Romans 8:37, "Nay, in all these things we are more than conquerors through him that loved us." It also says in Matthew 5:45 . . . "he maketh his sun to rise on the evil and on the good, and sendeth rain on the just and on the unjust." And so I wish for plenty of sunshine on all who've been showered upon, to help alleviate their symptoms of these syndromes once and for all through believing in prayer, faith and the word of God. After all, Jesus Christ is the Healer and he can heal any and all sicknesses and diseases.

Coming up from a semi-invalid and practically bedridden state all the way to fairly good health was a life changing experience for me. And now I have put the key that Jesus Christ gave me to unlocking the chains of darkness that these syndromes have caused into your hands. Now all you have to do is turn the key.

ACKNOWLEDGMENTS

I would like to acknowledge the Lord Jesus Christ and those in His Church who preach and teach the Holy Bible, including divine healing. I thank all who prayed for me. Again, I especially thank my wife who waited on me hand and foot, tirelessly massaging trigger points and spasms on a daily basis. Not to mention listening to complaints for years, putting up with irritability and helping nurture, as it were, a wounded soldier, back to health. I thank all of my family, including aunts and uncles, etc. for all of their encouragement, as well as countless physicians. Thanks to my computer programmers; Patricia Adcock and Cheryl Martin, agent, editor, Martha Griffin and publisher for helping me turn this book out. It's so wonderful when everyone plays their part. It's like a finely tuned orchestra at its best concert. Every sound is crisp and clear.

I am also grateful for the following publishers for allowing me to reprint parts of previously published material: Lipincott, Williams & Wilkins (LWW) for Illustrations by Travell and Simons, and the American College of Rheumatology's Arthritis and Rheumatism illustration's of Tender points and 1990 classification criteria for Fibromyalgia.

VGM's list of occupations.

All Illustrations by Thomas McAteer Studios.

INTRODUCTION

I tried desperately to get somebody else to write this book because I didn't want to and didn't know if I could do it or not. But after everybody turned me down and imposed that famous question "why don't you just write it yourself?" I finally decided to just write it myself. It's a privilege and an honor to share with you the latest medical Breakthroughs that I have discovered against these illnesses.

This book is different than other books because while the others talk all about the problem, this book promises a solution to the problem and delivers.

The truth is that people want an easy and effective way out of their illness and this is a simple program to follow and I believe it's the most effective natural remedy to date against these illnesses. This is a book of healing, encouragement, hope, faith, and most of all charity. It's about how I triumphed from sickness back to reasonable health, and am showing you how you may be able to do the same. Many books on these conditions have taught us many things, but none will ever push as close to healing these epidemics as this book will. This is a book which will move you from out of your seat to praying to God and believing for your own healing miracle. Only Jesus Christ and the Holy Bible is better for these illnesses. So sit back and absorb as much as you can. I'll show you all about these illnesses and then, of course, all about the remedy.

PART I

THE ILLNESSES

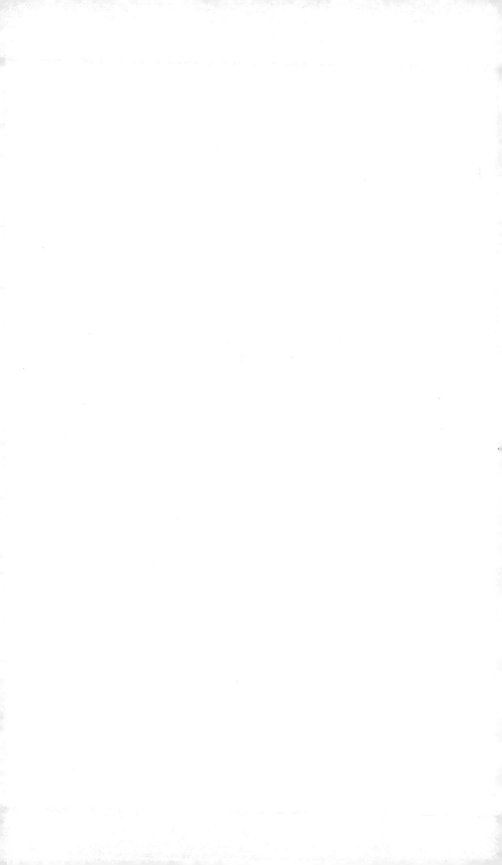

CHAPTER 1

Why Me?

Many times the question is asked, "Why me?" Why did this have to happen NOW? Some say they didn't really know but let me tell you of one account recorded in the Bible. In John 9:2-3, Jesus Christ saw a blind man and when the disciples asked him, "who did sin, this man, or his parents, that he was born blind?" Jesus answered, "neither, hath this man sinned nor his parents: but that the works of God should be made manifest in him." I'm sure this man asked "Why me?" many times throughout his entire life, and now he certainly knows why.

Jesus continued and spat on the ground, made spittle and anointed his eyes with it and commanded the man to go wash in the pool of Siloam (which means sent).

Much opposition came to this man and to Jesus Christ for the miracle that was done. Some people just can't stand it when a good thing like a miracle happens to someone else. They eventually pressed the man so much about who healed him that he ended up teaching all of those so-called teachers of the law that Jesus Christ is from God and also told them in John 9:32 "since the world began was it not heard that any man opened the eyes of one that was born blind." This was prophesied in Isaiah 35:4-5, saying that God himself would come and save us and open the eyes of the blind and the ears of the deaf that they might understand, both spiritually and naturally.

Let's understand something. Some people have brought sickness upon themselves, such as in some cases of AIDS, but there are those who didn't know better or are in no fault of their own, such as a man born blind or a sickness like FMS, MPS, CFS, CFIDS, GWS or AA of which no one even knows the causes and more less, the cures. We are definitely at the mercy of God. No matter how much we record and describe these illnesses, the bottom line is that nobody knows the exact causes at this time but God alone. And if you want out like the blind man did, go to God yourself. After you get healed, you'll be teaching others what's really going on just like the blind man taught the so-called teachers. Truly the first became last and the last became first. Did it not? This miraculous event can undoubtedly open the eyes of one's understanding to who the blind people really are.

In 1988, I was in college to study for a pre-med degree to prepare for medical school, hoping to become a doctor. During the first year I was struck down with FMS, MPS, CFS and AA. Whether one of them or all four of them is of no consequence, as you will see. But I didn't know exactly what it was and neither did my physicians. Contracting the illnesses, with me being stressed out in college with 18 hours and many other activities only exacerbated the anxiety that accompanies these syndromes. Though the first doctor I saw said I had a virus, the anxiety continued to perplex the other physicians so they deemed it strictly psychological (or better yet, psychiatrical); adding that this had nothing to do with my physical condition whatsoever.

Once the stigma of a psychiatric diagnosis was applied to me and recorded in medical records, it caused me to suffer many other misdiagnoses and mistreatments. And worse yet that hindered me from unveiling the true underlying diagnosis of FMS, MPS and/or CFS. It took several years to get to the bottom of the truth about that. Some of the first doctors missed tender points. They never bothered to look. I'd studied about many of these problems in psychology and it just wasn't adding up. I'd never hallucinated, as one physician stated in his records, but nevertheless I was drugged just as if I were. They didn't find trigger points either. They never looked, even though I did complain about the pain. Maybe they just didn't know what to look for. As one counselor put it, I was just a bowl of soup.

No matter how many times I told them I was hurting and even showing them with my finger the exact, specific points on my muscles where I was hurting, they just simply did not believe me. And then when they'd leave, I'd pray to the Lord and tell him all about how they would not believe me and I'd just cry from the unrelenting pain and anguish. They treated me like I was ignorant and knew nothing. I tried to contend only because I knew I wasn't telling any lies. I knew it wasn't all in my head like they were trying to force me to believe. These doctors never really listened to me, "the patient."

It took years to somehow get out of that vicious cycle and find a physician that amazingly listened to me "the patient" and went straight to the muscles that I was pointing to all along with his own hands and he easily felt trigger points all over my shoulders, neck and back. That was in 1991.

Finally, somebody believed me. He diagnosed Myofascial Pain Syndrome and said I had Fibromyalgia. I went through trigger point therapy and eventually I was discontinued from treatment, even though the trigger points persisted. I continued for years with constant pain and extreme fatigue and so many other symptoms as well. Eventually something was done about FMS as to making it a genuine illness by giving it a code in the 10th revision of the ICD (International Code of Diagnoses). The code is M79.0 (Consensus . . . , 1992).

Then it finally came to the point that I knew I needed to get more serious about this problem. I'd prayed many times before but this one particular time I was more determined than ever before to get an answer from God alone. So I got down on my knees and did some hard, serious praying, asking for complete deliverance and healing. I knew I wasn't going to stop praying until the Lord blessed me. After a very long time he gave me three special words. These three word's were lifechanging. As I learned to trust and believe him on those words over time he truly answered my prayers and brought them to pass. With God being sovereign as he is, he really didn't have to answer those prayers, but he did. And I'm so glad he did, too. As it is written in II Timothy 2:6, "The husbandman that laboureth must be first partaker of the fruits." I've certainly earned my degree from being ill with these syndromes. And regaining health is certainly graduation. Truly the works of God were manifested in my life and now that I'm healthier, I'm prescribing to others the same remedy that helped me. That's the answer to "Why me."

CHAPTER 2

Fibromyalgia

Fibromyalgia is a common painful condition or syndrome characterized by fatigue, non-restorative sleep, stiffness (especially in the morning), and widespread musculoskeletal pain in the muscles and other fibrous connective tissues (ligaments and tendons) (Consensus . . . , 1992). See the consensus document on Fibromyalgia.

Experts have given the term Fibromyalgia to a group of signs and symptoms to help classify it from other illnesses. (A syndrome is a collection of signs and symptoms characterizing a particular disease or condition. A sign is what a physician finds upon his/her examination. A symptom is what you tell your physician). Some believe that FMS is a type of neurotransmitter dysfunction rather than a neuromuscular condition, such as MPS (Starlanyl . . . , 1996).

The word Fibromyalgia broken down gives a more precise description of its characteristics. "Fibro: means "fiber or fibrous tissue," "my" means "muscle," and "algia" means "painful condition of."

"Fibromyalgia" is much more accurate in description than some of the other names that have been commonly used, such as, "Fibrositis" and other "-itis" names which indicate that inflammation is present, because inflammation is not a significant finding in Fibromyalgia (Arthritis Foundation, 1998). See the following list of other names used to describe Fibromyalgia.

The Many Names of Fibromyalgia

Anxiety Neurosis	Neurocirculatory Asthenia
Cerviobrachial Syndrome	Neurofibrositis
Chronic Nervous Exhaustion	Nodular Rheumatism
Chronic Pain Syndrome	Nonrestorative Sleep Syndrome
Chronic Rheumatism	Occupation Cerviobrachial Disorder
Cumulative Trauma Disorders	Occupational Myalgia
Fat Herniations	Occupational Overuse Syndrome
Fibromyositis	Pain Amplification Syndrome
Fibropathic Syndrome	Piriformis Syndrome
Functional Myopathy	Pressure Point Syndrome
Hypersensitive Areas	Primary Fibrositis
Interstitial Myofibromyositis	Psychogenic Rheumatism
Lesion Areas Low Back Syndrome	Repetitive Strain Injury
Muscle Callus	Repetitive Strain Syndrome
Muscle Gelling	Rheumatic Myositis
Muscle Hardening	Rheumatic Myopathy
Muscular Rheumatism	Rheumatic Myositis
Musculofascial Pain	Rheumatic Pain Modulation Disorder
Muskelharte	Scapulocostal Syndrome
Muskelschweile	Sensitive Areas
Myalgia	Sensitive Deposits
Myodysneuria	Soft Tissue Rheumatism
Myofascial Pain Dysfunction	Splanchnic Neurasthenia
Myofascial Pain Syndrome	Tension Fibrositis of the legs
Myofascitis	Tension Myalgia
Myofibrositis	Tension Myalgia of the pelvic floor
Myogelose	Tension Neck
Myopathia E. Labore	Traumatic Myofibrositis
Myositis	Traumatic Neurosis
Myospastic Syndrome	Trigger Point Syndrome
Nerve Point Syndrome	Trigger Zone Syndrome

Figure 2-1: From Chronic Muscle Pain Syndrome Paul Davidson, M.D.

Some of the names used to diagnose fibromyalgia such as "Myofascial Pain Syndrome," may have been used interchangeably with "Fibromyalgia" to actually describe the same syndrome. Although some hold the opinion that MPS and Fibromyalgia are different syndromes, others believe that they are one and the same, especially when considering that these two syndromes have very similar signs and symptoms.

What FMS Affects

FMS mainly affects fibrous connective tissue including ligaments, tendons, cartilage and muscles, mostly where muscles join to tendons and attach to bones (Eichner, 1990; Arthritis Foundation, 1998). It is non-articular (not occurring in the joints) and it is considered to be a form of muscular rheumatism, since that refers to aches, pains and stiffness associated with muscles and other connective tissues (Arthritis Foundation, 1998; Eichner, 1990).

It usually affects the muscles all over the body: hips, thighs, arms, legs, neck, head, upper back, lower back, shoulders, chest and abdominal muscles. The involvement of the Frontalis, Occipitalis, and Temporalis muscles (muscles of the head) could help to explain most tension headaches.

Theoretically, the muscle of the heart, lungs (especially diaphragm) and smooth muscles of the intestinal tract are affected as well. Hence, panic attacks (tachycardia), IBS (Irritable Bowel Syndrome) and hyperventilation, just to name a few obvious signs and symptoms.

FMS seems to cause patients to be in a type of de-conditioning state. They just seem to get out of physical shape very easily.

Most of those affected with FMS are women and women are built for endurance more than men are. They give birth to children and carry children around all day in their arms and still have energy left over. Women also typically outlive men by sometimes as much as ten years.

The sleeping pattern for most FMS patients is affected as well by the disruption of Stage IV sleep (the deepest stage) which seems to be vital for muscle restoration (Eichner, 1990; Arthritis Foundation, 1998). Hence, fatigue, forgetfulness, anxiety and depression.

NON-RESTORATIVE SLEEP

Electroencephalographic tests have shown evidence that there is alpha-wave (wakefulness) intrusion into the deep slower delta-wave (Stage IV, a.k.a. nonrapid eye movement [NREM]) sleep as well as other sleep stages (Krsnich-Shriwise, 1997). Fibromyalgia patients experience about 60% of alpha-wave intrusion of stage IV sleep while patients with insomnia and dysthymia experience about 25% (Krsnich-Shriwise, 1997).

However, after this program, you will be getting deeper sleep allowing you to literally get back to dreaming again.

FIBROFOG

Fibrofog is a term given to the feeling of fogginess in the cognitive process of memory and/or concentration usually secondary to FMS.

The cognitive deficits seem to be least bothersome while going through this program. And even after stopping this program, the fibrofog was virtually non-existent for me.

Signs and Symptoms of FMS

The American College of Rheumatology (ACR) has posted a fine benchmark of signs and symptoms to help meet the diagnostic criteria for FMS (listed below).

Symptoms of Fibromyalgia

- Tenderness of at least 11 of 18 specific anatomical points
- Stiffness, especially in A.M. upon awakening
- Sleep disturbances/insomnia
- Chronic aching
- Pain
- Anxiety
- Depression
- Chronic fatigue
- Gastrointestinal disturbances
- Irritable bowel syndrome
- Subjective soft tissue swelling
- Cardiovascular problems (dizziness, palpitations)
- Muscle spasms and trigger points/muscle jerking
- Fluid retention
- Poor memory
- PMS
- Tightening sensations

Figure 2-2: With permission from the American College of Rheumatology 1990 Classification Criteria.

In addition to that list, there are other symptoms occasionally associated with Fibromyalgia.

Other Symptoms Occasionally Associated with Fibromyalgia

- Generalized/migraine headaches that can last for years
- Flu-like Symptoms
- Frequent sore throat
- Painful lymph node in armpits/neck

- Impaired concentration
- Sensitivity to weather changes
- Radiating pain that moves from joint to joint without swelling or redness
- TMJ
- Jaw and facial tenderness
- Numbness/tingling sensations
- Dry eyes/mouth
- Irregular breathing rhythm, shortness of breath, pulmonary function
- Sensitivity to light and noise (phono/photosensitivity), foods
- Teeth grinding at night
- Hypo/Hyperglycemia
- Ulcers
- High/Low Blood Pressure
- Asthma/Allergies
- Bursitis
- Seizures
- Anxiety (Panic) Attacks
- Circulatory Problems
- Thoracic Outlet Syndrome (TOS)
- Poor circulation/cold feet/Raynaud's phenomenon
- Sinus problems
- Thyroid disorder
- Muscle weakness (myasthenia like symptoms)
- Sleep problems/Apnea
- Reduced tolerance for exercise
- Restless arms and legs
- Ptosis (eyelid drooping)
- Carpal Tunnel Syndrome (CTS)
- Irritable Bladder and/or Urinary Tract Infections (UTI)
- Urinary burning/urgency/frequency
- Mitral valve prolapse (MVP)
- Gastroesophageal Reflux Disease (GERD)
- Impotency
- Post polio syndrome (PPS)
- CFS (a.k.a. CFIDS or ME)
- Immune system deficiency/abnormalities
- Water retention
- Lab tests are negative despite feeling very ill
- Pain in connective tissues (muscles, tendons, cartilage and ligaments)
- All 4 quadrants of the body have pain
- Hypersensitive skin, itching/burning

- Coordination impairment
- Chest pain/pressure
- Symptoms exacerbated by physical/emotional stress
- Intermittent hearing difficulties, especially low frequencies

(Williamson, 1996; various sources)

What Are Tender Points?

Tender points are places in soft tissue that hurt when they are pressed upon and do not refer pain elsewhere (Starlanyl . . . , 1996). They are located in specific points on the body and usually occur bilaterally. The following diagram shows the typical pattern for tender points in FMS but are not limited to these areas only because they can occur elsewhere due to other illness (es) and/or injury (ies).

The American College of Rheumatology 1990 criteria for the classification of fibromyalgia

History of widespread pain has been present for at least three months.
Definition: Pain is widespread when all of the following are present:

- Pain in both sides of the body
- Pain above and below the waist

In addition, axial skeletal pain (cervical spine, anterior chest, thoracic spine or low back pain) must be present. Low back pain is considered lower segment pain.
Pain in 11 of 18 tender point sites on digital palpation.
Definition: Pain, on digital palpation, must be present in at least 11 of the following 18 tender point sites:

- *Occiput* (2)—at the suboccipital muscle insertions
- *Low cervical* (2)—at the anterior aspects of the intertransverse spaces at C5-C7
- *Trapezius* (2)—at the midpoint of the upper border
- *Supraspinatus* (2)—at origins, above the scapula spine near the medial border
- *Second rib* (2)—upper lateral to the second costochondral junction
- *Lateral epicondyle* (2)—2 cm distal to the epicondyles
- *Gluteal* (2)—in upper outer quadrants of buttocks in anterior fold of muscle
- *Greater trochanter* (2)—posterior to the trochanteric prominence
- *Knee* (2)—at the medial fat pad proximal to the joint line

Digital palpation should be performed with an approximate force of 4 kg. A tender point has to be painful at palpation, not just "tender" (Reprinted with permission from the American College of Rheumatology (ACR), 1990).

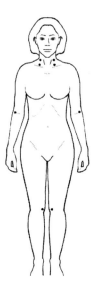

Figure 2-3: Location of tender points: Front (ACR, 1990)

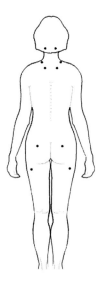

Figure 2-4: Location of tender points: Back (ACR, 1990).

What causes Tender Points?

Some experts believe that the neurotransmitter dysfunction causes connective tissue to become stiff, tight and even shortened (Starlanyl . . . , 1996). This then constrains the rate at which nutrition, water and oxygen are exchanged on the cellular level, therefore causing waste build-up. The area is now trying to guard itself from further pain, and tenses up, involuntarily producing a tender point. These tender points can back up the cell rate exchange then turning into a trigger point. This process can also reverse itself as well (Starlanyl . . . , 1996).

Diagnosing FMS

FMS can be diagnosed by widespread musculoskeletal pain and also having 11 out of 18 tender points. This definition is being used to help standardize research protocols (Consensus . . . , 1992; American College of Rheumatology, 1990).

Despite these definitions, currently there are no tests or x-rays which can determine an absolute diagnosis of FMS (See Figure 2-3 and 2-4).

Type of Physician to see for diagnosis

Rheumatologists are the physicians who specialize in disorders of the joints and muscles. Find one that is well trained in locating trigger points and tender points (one who believes and understands that this is not an imaginary illness and will help rule out illnesses of psychogenic origin) in order to get properly diagnosed.

Moreover, it is only wise on your part to get checked out physically before accepting an emotional or psychiatric diagnosis as your primary illness, especially when realizing that anxiety and depression are more than likely the result of having FMS rather than the cause of it.

Prognosis of FMS

The prognosis of FMS is poor. Even though most patients have chronic symptoms, many do eventually resume increased activities with treatment. Most importantly is that FMS is not progressive and objective findings do not develop (Tierney, Jr., McPhee, Papadakis, 1998).

Treatment of FMS

The most commonly prescribed treatment is the combination of drug therapy and physical therapy. Tricyclic antidepressants are often prescribed to help induce stage IV sleep and to help alleviate depression.

Anxiety agents are sometimes prescribed to help ease tension, anxiety and muscle twitching.

Muscle relaxants are prescribed as well to help give a relaxing effect which also helps to induce sleep. Flexaril has been commonly prescribed for these symptoms.

Narcotic pain killers are being prescribed to help patients deal with their pain. On the contrary, however, NSAID pain relievers do not seem to be very effective.

There are many drugs being prescribed to help with every symptom known to man and they even help in those situations, but today's physicians do not have a single drug to treat and relieve all of the symptoms of FMS, MPS, CFS, CFIDS or GWS simultaneously.

Physical therapy is prescribed to help with almost every aspect of FMS. It helps stimulate endorphins (the brain's natural pain killers) and relax muscles as well as strengthen the immune system, just to name a few.

Aerobic exercise and stretching exercise have been what physicians have been prescribing. They are supposed to help strengthen the body and even encourage proper posture. Heat, especially moist heat, is helpful to painful areas on the body. Gentle massage is soothing and relaxing and even helps stimulate endorphins as well. In today's medical community though, these treatments were to be ongoing indefinitely. Even still, there are many other non-medical treatments which are practiced by patients today.

CHAPTER 3

Myofascial Pain Syndrome

Myofascial Pain Syndrome (MPS) is considered a common but non-articular rheumatic condition characterized by pain, tenderness, and stiffness in the muscles and other connective tissues. It is not the same as Fibromyalgia. It is also considered a neuromuscular disorder. Aside from pain and stiffness, the main feature of MPS is the presence of trigger points (Berkow & Fletcher, 1987). Trigger points are hard, built-up waste places in muscles that hurt to the touch, and also refer pain elsewhere in the body (Starlanyl . . . , 1996). Unlike tender points in FMS, which hurt only at those points where pressed upon without referring the pain elsewhere (Starlanyl . . . , 1996). It has been thought that activity and stress aggravate symptoms of MPS. It is given the name Myofascial Pain Syndrome because the pain is mostly in the muscles ("myo") fascia. Fascia is the connective tissue that is found throughout the entire body which helps to surround muscles as well as other tissues to help protect and support them.

Rheumatologists are the specialists of choice to see when choosing a doctor for treatment, but first inquire if the doctor of your choice is knowledgeable in properly diagnosing and treating this condition.

Diagnosis is made based on the presence of widespread musculoskeletal pain and trigger points.

These trigger points are taut bands of muscle fibers and have a "ropy" feeling to the touch and cause a "jump sign" which is an involuntary shortening of the fibrous muscle band when palpated (Fomby and Mellion, 1997). Trigger points are classified as being either active or latent. The active trigger points cause constant or persistent pain while latent trigger points go unnoticed until they are palpated (Fomby . . . , 1997). When trigger points are palpated they not only hurt where they are pressed upon but also refer pain to another area on the body, called the "reference zone." These zones are not only predictable but are consistent and are usually distal (which is away from where they are palpated) (Fomby . . . , 1997).

Both active and latent trigger points create a jump sign when palpated and may also affect the muscle group by weakness, range of motion, and ability to stretch actively and passively. (Fomby . . . , 1997.) Due to increased stress to the involved muscle groups, active trigger points can activate what is called "satellite" or secondary trigger points in the reference zone (Fomby . . . , 1997).

A main problem with trigger points is that there is a starving for food and oxygen with accumulated waste at the affected areas (Starlanyl . . . , 1996). Some reasons thought to cause trigger points are:

- Overuse
- Repetitive motion trauma
- Bruises
- Strains
- Joint problems
- Surgery
- Auto accident
- Slip and falls
  (Starlanyl . . . , 1996)

There is also combined conditions of FMS and MPS called the FMS/MPS complex. This is where you have both conditions at the same time.

There is currently no x-ray or blood test that can help substantiate the diagnosis of MPS. Most of the tests taken are used to rule out other disorders.

The prognosis for MPS seems to be favorable when realizing that trigger points can disappear spontaneously. But they can reappear under stressful conditions and can also become chronic.

Treatment for MPS has often been reduced stress levels, physical therapy, massage, gentle stretching exercises, medication to help with sleep and even injections at areas of focal tenderness (Berkow . . . , 1987). Cryotherapy (excessive cold), relaxation and biofeedback have also been used.

There is currently no medicine that can cure MPS according to the medical community. However, Travell and Simons (1992) found that Potaba™ medication did help to ease the tightness in the myofascia. (Personally, I've not tried this medication). Most MPS patients were informed that they could get rid of most of the pain from trigger points, but not the trigger points themselves. But now with this program you can get rid of the trigger points as well as the pain associated with them. Could this program then be an outright cure for MPS?

In massage treatments, nurses and/or physical therapists use thumbs to press and hold on the trigger points. They say that this will stop the blood flow and allow the trigger points and muscles to relax. They even use their elbows on large trigger points. (I've even had my wife use her heels and knees in some places. See illustrations for trigger point locations).

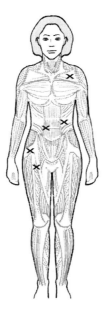

Figure 3-1: Trigger Points of the Front.

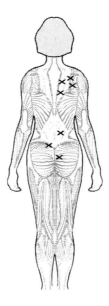

Figure 3-2: Trigger Points of the Back.

Trigger points may appear in other places than those that are illustrated because every patient is uniquely different.

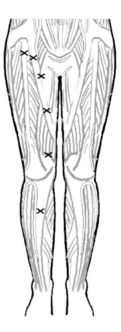

Figure 3-3: Trigger Points of the Front of the Legs

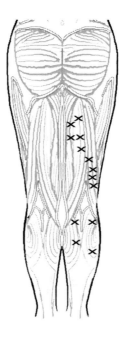

Figure 3-4: Trigger Points of the Back of the Legs.

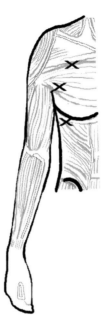

Figure 3-5: Trigger Points of the Front of the Arms.

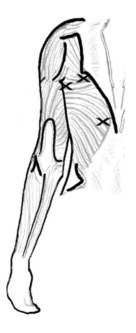

Figure 3-6: Trigger Points of the Back of the Arms.

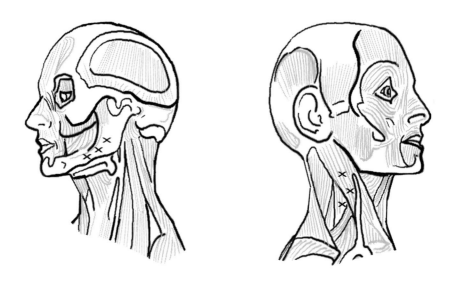

Figure 3-7: Trigger Points of the Front of the Neck

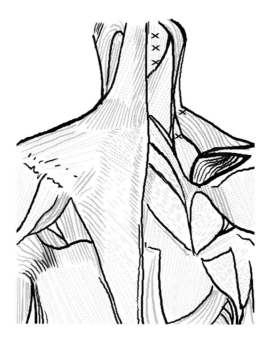

Figure 3-8: Trigger Points of the Back of the Neck

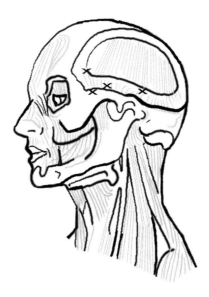

Figure 3-9: Trigger Points of the Side of the Head.

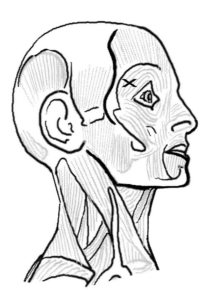

Figure 3-10: Trigger Points of the Face.

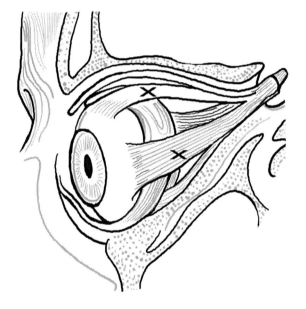

Figure 3-11: Trigger Points of the Extrinsic eye muscles.

CHAPTER 4

Chronic Fatigue Syndrome
(a.k.a. CFIDS or ME)

Chronic Fatigue Syndrome is a syndrome whose main sign is fatigue for 6 months or more. CFS is estimated to affect 2.5 million Americans or more, mostly women. Some believe that CFS is the exact same illness as FMS, while others disagree.

CFS is also sometimes called chronic fatigue immune dysfunction syndrome or CFIDS. People may still have chronic fatigue syndrome even if no tender points or trigger points are present. In some countries it is also known as myalgic encephalomyelitis or ME.

CFS seems to affect the nervous system although no specific tests can prove or disprove its presence. Some signs and symptoms are:

- Fatigue
- Exhaustion
- Low grade fever
- Sore throat
- Chills/night sweats
- Swollen/tender lymph nodes
- Muscle weakness
- Muscle aches/pains
- Headache
- Painful joints
- Allergic reactions
- Weight gain or loss
- Skin rashes
- Feeling of inability to exercise
- Anxiety/depression

General fatigue is the feeling of exhaustion, weakness or tiredness which makes regular tasks seem impossible. Ohayon and Shapiro (2000) list four basic types of fatigue:

(1) Objective fatigue is the type you feel when you are not able to maintain a certain level of effort during exercise.

(2) Subjective fatigue is the fatigue you feel which suppresses the desire to even engage in exercise.

(3) Systemic fatigue is fatigue seen in athletes who have sustained a prolonged physical effort.

(4) Asthenia or neurasthenia fatigue is general weakness, tiredness or exhaustion without physiological abnormalities after exercise and frequently accompanied in patients with poor sleep complaints (Ohayon and Shapiro, 2000).

The first three are thought to be of neuromuscular origin, whereas the last is considered a state of mind (Ohayon . . . , 2000). Fatigue can be caused by a number of things such as rheumatic diseases, arthritis, lupus, FMS, MPS, emotional stress, any illness, depression, joint pain, pain, any stress, poor sleep habits, anemia, lack of exercise or even too much exercise (Managing your Fatigue, 1997). Fatigue can make you feel so tired that you have no energy at all. It can make you feel like you have increased pain, a lack of concentration, irritability and even like you have lost control of your life (Managing your Fatigue, 1997).

General practitioners and internists are usually the first to see, but if symptoms persist, request to see a rheumatologist who is well-trained in FMS and MPS, one who can spot and differentiate between trigger points and tender points in case you may have FMS or MPS as well.

CFS is diagnosed by having fatigue that persists for 6 months or more and having some of the other symptoms with it. A newly revised definition of CFS was published in 1994 by the U.S. Center of Disease Control or (CDC), stating that fatigue must be present for 6 months or more while also having 4 of the following 8 symptoms:

- Substantial impairment in short-term memory or concentration
- Sore throat
- Tender lymph nodes
- Muscle pain
- Multi-joint pain without swelling or redness
- Headaches of a new type, pattern or severity
- Unrefreshing sleep
- Post-exertional malaise lasting more than 24 hours
  (CFIDS Research, 2001)

The prognosis of CFS is not so favorable but some people seem to do better after 2 years. The first year seems to be the most gruesome. The most commonly prescribed treatments are anti-anxiety medicines, anti-depressants (mostly to help with getting better sleep and chronic pain) and other experimental measures. The not-so-good news is that, according to most physicians, the treatment may be indefinite. As with FMS and MPS, there is no known cure for CFS outside of getting relief from the remedy offered in this book. Furthermore, like FMS and MPS, there are no laboratory tests or x-rays to confirm the diagnosis of CFS.

If you've ever had the flu (especially the flu of the year 1999-2000 that swept the U.S.) and then felt that long, lingering fatigue that followed, then you'll have a good idea of what CFS really feels like. Only imagine feeling that fatigue persistently year after year. Dr. Crook of Jackson, Tennessee, the author of The Yeast Connection, once said on a television interview that the males born in Portsmouth, VA have the highest percentage rate of Chronic Fatigue Syndrome than any other city in the U.S. (By the way, that's the very city where I was born).

Furthermore, when I was in my thirties, a rheumatologist in a different state diagnosed that I had had FMS since I was a child. I grew up in Norfolk, VA. And once when I was about 8 or 9 years old I became very ill with a fever of 103°-104°. I was burning up and felt like a red hot pepper. I was so fatigued during that illness that when I stood up to go to the rest room, I was faint, my vision would go black, and I would have to hold onto the walls until I could see again and proceed. The naval physicians diagnosed it as a virus. The rheumatologist I saw later felt that this was the start of FMS for me.

Many physicians are blaming CFS, a.k.a. CFIDS, a.k.a. ME, as "all in your head," as is often the case with FMS and/or MPS. However, there was an article written by Russell Lane (2000) titled "Chronic Fatigue Syndrome: Is it physical?" in the journal of neurology, neurosurgery and psychiatry abstracting a different article of a study done by Fulcher and White (2000). That study showed that CFS was not "all in your head." In fact, there was some physical evidence to show that there was a marked difference between the CFS patients and those not diagnosed with CFS. It was concluded in the following manner: sixty-six outpatients were recruited through a fatigue clinic at a general hospital department of psychiatry. They all agreed to participate in a trial of graded exercise therapy. Thirty healthy but sedentary controls were recruited and fifteen patients with major depression were recruited. The study divided the outpatients into the following categories in order to conduct the study:

- CFS patients
- Depressed patients
- Sedentary controls

All of the patients performed gradual aerobic exercise on treadmills. The study showed that the CFS patients compared to the sedentary controls were physically weaker, had a significantly reduced exercise capacity and also perceived greater effort during exercise and were equally unfit.

When compared with the depressed patients, the CFS patients had significantly higher submaximal oxygen uptake during exercise and perceived greater physical fatigue and incapacity.

The CFS group had lower peak oxygen consumption, lower maximal heart rates and lower plasma lactate concentrations than the sedentary controls. The greatest difference found was that the CFS group had a significantly weaker measurement of quadricep muscle strength when tested. This may also help us give face to the deconditioning that takes place in CFS patients. This is the first study that showed that there was a physical weakness in CFS patients. The physical therapy seemed to help all of the patients overall (Fulcher . . . , 2000). This is why the remedy in this book will help to minimize the fatigue. Lane (2000) concludes his article by saying that "whatever the mechanisms underlying 'fatigue,' exercise therapy is likely to become an increasingly important therapeutic modality in various fields and particularly in the management of chronic fatigue syndromes." This will apply to all chronic fatigue syndromes as well as to GWS, since chronic fatigue is one of the most prevalent symptoms. This may also include Anxiety (panic) Attacks.

Many scientists have studied CFS but maybe not in the most effective areas to gather the best data that will help patients get to the ultimate place they long to be, which is a "firm or legitimate diagnosis." Just having that is a first major step. The patients are only seeking the truth to their complaints whether physiological, psychiatric, or both. Doctors offer sympathy and maybe some symptomatic relief but nothing close to 100% cure. In Clarke's (2000) published article in *Social Work in Healthcare*, 2000, it states that when it comes to CFS "effective treatment protocols are elusive," and "causal factors are unclear" (Clarke, 2000). In Ohayon and Shapiro's (2000) article, they further delved into the study of whether sleep disturbances cause CFS or CFS causes sleep disturbances, and concluded that no definitive conclusions can be drawn at this time. The article goes on to explain that in some cases sleep disturbances would have negated the diagnosis of CFS, yet in other cases sleep disturbance may have increased fatigue. Ohayon and Shapiro (2000) continue saying that many CFS patients either nap in the day or spend some time in bed. They say that this may aggravate the sleep disturbances and lead to more daytime fatigue.

All of this they say is a vicious cycle that may help contribute to the chronicity of the fatigue. Especially since it will lead to further neuromuscular deconditioning and even other fatigue mechanisms like:

- Arthritis
- Headache or migraine
- Epilepsy
- Obesity
- Heart disease

- Parkinson's disease
- Head injury
- Cerebromuscular disease
- Viral or bacterial infection
- Food allergy
- Huntington's disease
- Dystonia
- Ataxia
- Dyskinesia
- Spastic torticollis
- Cancer
- Hyper or hypothyroidism
- Multiple sclerosis
- Dementia
- Gastrointestinal illness
- And end organ failure, e.g., liver, renal or respiratory failure (Ohayon . . . , 2000)

The program outlined in this book may help reduce insomnia and other sleep problems associated with fatigue. Yes, it's true, further conclusive studies are needed, but there are some new breakthroughs that are helping us to understand CFS better. So before you give up and throw in the towel, give this program a chance to help you get out of the vicious cycle of CFS. You just might get the help you've been searching and waiting for.

CHAPTER 5

Gulf War Syndrome

On January 16, 1991 the United States of America declared war on the country of Iraq. Iraq had invaded and was taking over Kuwait and was also setting their sites on Saudi Arabia and other neighboring countries to take control of the world's oil supply. Kuwait helps to supply a strong percentage of the world's oil. So, the threat of Kuwait being overthrown was of critical importance to the U.S. The U.S. began to deploy ships, planes, artillery and troops (about 697,000) to the Persian Gulf. The U.S. called these operations "Desert Storm" and "Desert Shield."

The threat of Iraq using biological or chemical warfare agents was very real to the U.S., or at least the Pentagon claimed that it was. Even so, the threat was still possible and the troops were given vaccination shots to help them ward off attacks of these types of weapons, including shots to counter anthrax and botulism.

The war ended quickly and is one of the shortest wars on record, just 44 days. Iraq vacated Kuwait and surrendered. Some of their troops composed of just teenagers with warfare weapons. In the end Kuwait was liberated and now still has control over their oil fields. The United States' casualties were minimal (but not to go unrecognized) compared to Iraq's.

Then the U.S. troops started coming home and began to have mysterious multiple signs and symptoms. It was suggested they were victims of biological or chemical warfare. Since that time, many have sought medical attention and have even gone through many tests to help find the exact cause of their condition, but mostly to no decisive conclusion. Some experts believe that they have been exposed while others do not. So, for the sake of preventing further arguments, we'll assume that the veterans probably have been exposed to some kind of agent(s) whether chemical, biological, natural or at least have a unique syndrome (cluster of symptoms) worth recognizing. We'll call it the Gulf War Syndrome. The Gulf War Syndrome is a term used to describe these veterans with unexplained illnesses, often characterized by discomfort, symptoms of which are listed below. According to the American Legion (Gulf War Syndrome, 2001) these are the following symptoms for Gulf War Syndrome:

- Chronic fatigue
- Signs and symptoms involving skin (including skin rashes and unusual hair loss)
- Headache
- Muscle pain (myalgia)
- Neurologic signs and symptoms (nervous system disorders which could manifest themselves as numbness in one's arm, for instance)
- Neuropsychological signs or symptoms (including memory loss)
- Signs or symptoms involving upper or lower respiratory system
- sleep disturbances
- Gastrointestinal signs or symptoms (including diarrhea or constipation)
- Cardiomuscular signs or symptoms
- Menstrual disorders

Other symptoms not on this list may include:

- Running nose
- Urinary urgency
- twitching
- Sores
- Joint pain
  (various sources)

GWS has many of the same symptoms as FMS, MPS and CFS. Chronic fatigue is one of the most prevalent symptoms in these presumably with Gulf War Syndrome. The Gulf War veterans also "experienced a wide variety of physical and environmental exposures as well as psychological and emotional traumas during their service in the Gulf" (Hunt, 1999).

Many of the vets were thought to have post-traumatic stress disorder (PTSD) since some vets did see casualties, combat and may have had beliefs that they had been exposed to chemical or biological agents. However, in the Journal of Occupational and Environmental Medicine, Pamela Kaires (1999) cites that "Roberta White, a Boston clinical neuropsychologist with more than 30 papers published on environmental and occupational toxin exposure stated that the health symptoms of Gulf War veterans could not be fully explained by post-traumatic stress disorder status or other psychiatric diagnoses." There are other theories as to why these veterans are experiencing these symptoms like: "exposure to low levels of chemical agents; an unusual chronic infective disease; exposure to biologic warfare agents; side effects of vaccines or medications administered to Gulf War participants; or some combination of these factors" (Frequently Asked Questions, 2001).

Most of the symptoms that the Gulf War veterans have presented in clinics "bring to mind other conditions that similarly elude current medical understanding—

fibromyalgia, chronic fatigue syndrome, multiple chemical sensitivities (MCS), as well as many common conditions with psychophysiologic components (hyperacidity/peptic ulcer disease, irritable bowel syndrome, musculoskeletal/tension/vascular headaches)" (Hunt, 1999). While proponents of the Gulf War Syndrome are accused of being hungry for money through any means of litigation from the U.S. government or even the Iraqi government, nobody is getting down to the nitty and gritty of helping these veterans and others who have GWS get healed of their symptoms and complaints. Most believe that these vets are not making up most of their symptoms. In fact, in a study by McCauley, et al. (1999), there was only a 70% participation rate in the 454 vets who were eligible for the study to help determine the cause of their signs and symptoms. Work responsibilities were the most frequent reason given for those not participating. On top of that, of all their survey responders, 90% of those that did participate (vets in the Oregon and Washington area) have gone on to either full-time or part-time work despite their symptoms. When weighing all of the evidence, one would have to conclude that these veterans are not malingerers, to say the least. On January 8, 1997, Dr. Robert Haley, chief of epidemiology at UT Southwestern Medical Center in Dallas, along with other researchers, came to a conclusion that "Gulf War veterans are suffering from three primary syndromes indicating brain and nerve damage caused by wartime exposure to combinations of low-level nerve agents and other common chemicals" (UT Southwestern Team, 1997). This was a major breakthrough. Haley and colleagues are the first to show a neuroscientific basis for the cause of Gulf War Syndrome (Rosenberg, 2000). In a series of articles published in JAMA, 1997 by Haley and colleagues, as well as the Iowa Persian Gulf Study Group (Rosenberg, 2000), showed that these researchers presented evidence of 6 symptoms of a Persian Gulf War (PGW) syndrome (a.k.a. Gulf War Syndrome/GWS). They fall into the following subtypes:

(1) Impaired cognition;
(2) Confusion—ataxia;
(3) Arthromyoneuropathy;
(4) Phobia apraxia;
(5) Fever adenopathy; and
(6) Weakness and incontinence.

Rosenberg (2000) says that "comprehensive neuropsychological testing, brainstem auditory evoked potential and other detailed neurophysiological test results were abnormal in Gulf War veterans compared with control subjects." Rosenberg (2000) quotes "The observations by Haley and colleagues are a major advance in defining the neurological basis and cause of this perplexing and elusive complex of symptoms and findings." Another note about the Gulf War Syndrome is that some believe that it may have been caused by having consumed diet drinks, which contain aspartame, in hot weather (Operation Mission Impossible, 2001). In the article titled "Operation

Mission Impossible" (1994-2001) it is stated that the aspartame in diet sodas is a chemical poison and is composed of three components: aspartic acid, phenylalanine and a methyl ester. It also states that the methyl ester converts to methanol, which is wood alcohol, which is considered a severe metabolic poison. When this is in your body, the wood alcohol converts to formaldehyde, then to boric acid (which is ant sting poison). (Who wants to drink that?) The phenylalanine further breaks down into DKP, which is a brain tumor agent. So could this be yet the reason for the Gulf War Syndrome that is seen? Also, many of the Gulf War veterans' children have even been born with defects. There certainly may be a connection between the Gulf War and these babies' abnormalities. Abnormalities like heart defects, birth defects, spina-bifida, internal organ problems and many more, to name just a few. There also seems to be strong suspicions that there is a possible government cover-up when looking into these matters. The Department of Defense (DOD) persistently rejects that these veterans' illnesses could be linked to exposure from either chemical or biological weapons. Gulf War vets can apply for VA compensation as well as Social Security Disability if their illness disables them from being gainfully employed. There have been some treatments such as using doxycycline (anti-biotic medication) to help the GWS victims. However it has not become mainstream, probably because it doesn't cease all of the symptoms to a strong enough degree. Currently, there is no known cure for GWS as with FMS, MPS, and CFS.

Whether you believe that there is a true Gulf War Syndrome or not, these people are still suffering, and some type of effective treatment must be made available, and soon. In this book I've taken the "So we are here, now what?" approach. There is nothing that can be done to change the past; we can only take the problem that is here now, and work toward a plausible, safe and effective approach to get to a cure, treatment or remedy; one that will be the most effective without further invasive insults to the body and it's components through additional chemicals, whether in the form of vaccinations, medications or any other substance that is not organic and safe. The Remedy in this book offers just such a program that helps without the use of medications, with side effects or further neurological damage.

CHAPTER 6

Anxiety (Panic) Attacks

Imagine that you are driving down the road in your car and suddenly you feel extreme panic. Adrenaline rushes through your blood and your heart begins to pound like it's coming out of your chest. Your body is in its fight or flight state—a state where your brain produces powerful endorphins and supernatural strength. Your breathing becomes erratic and short, and you're feeling terrified even though there is no true outside threat to cause you to feel this way. You feel like you're having a heart attack and you perceive that you may really be having one. So, you call on the cell phone to 911 as you pull off the road and when they finally get to examine you they inform you that you've just had a panic attack. The heart attack that you thought you were having is a false alarm. Thank God. But the Anxiety (Panic) Attack you've just had is very real. The medics give you a tranquilizer and you calm down and everything feels close to normal again. You are released and you go home. The errand you were running is no longer important anymore. Who cares what you were doing or where you were going. The medics also handed you a piece of paper advising you to seek some type of medical attention.

OK. But what's causing this? Did you know that you may have another underlying illness bringing on these anxiety or panic attacks? Here are some other medical conditions that can present themselves as panic disorder (Merritt, 2000):

- Thyroid dysfunction
- Parathyroid dysfunction
- Adrenal dysfunction
- Vestibular dysfunction
- Seizure disorders
- Cerebrovascular events
- CNS stimulant intoxication
- CNS depressant withdrawal
- Cardiac disorders
- Hypoglycemia

In addition to that, panic attacks are not uncommon with FMS, MPS, CFS or even GWS.

What are panic attacks? "Panic attacks are discrete episodes of abrupt onset of intense fear accompanied by at least four symptoms of physiologic arousal." (Reprinted with permission from the Diagnostic and Statistical Manual of Mental Disorders, Fourth Edition, ©1994 American Psychiatric Association (DSM-IV):

- Palpitations, pounding heart, or accelerated heart beat
- Sweating
- Trembling or shaking
- Sensations of shortness of breath or smothering
- Feelings of choking
- Chest pain or discomfort
- Nausea or abdominal distress
- Feeling dizzy, unsteady, lightheaded or faint
- Derealization (feelings of unreality) or depersonalization (being detached from oneself)
- Fear of losing control or going crazy
- Fear of dying
- Paresthesias (numbness or tingling)
- Chills or hot flashes

In addition to these is:

- Terror—a sense that something horrible is about to happen and you are powerless to prevent it

Other conditions that may accompany panic disorder are (Hendrix, 1993):

- Simple phobias
- Social phobias
- Depression
- Obsessive-compulsive disorder (OCD)
- Alcohol abuse
- Drug abuse
- Suicidal tendencies
- Irritable bowel syndrome, and,
- Mitral valve prolapse

According to the National Institute of Mental Health (NIMH) there are approximately 3 million or more adults suffering with, or who will have, panic disorder in their lifetime in the United States (Hendrix, 1993). According to Paluska et al. (2000) anxiety disorders are grouped into 2 distinct categories: state anxiety or trait anxiety. State anxiety is an acute, transient psychological response to an event or stimulus and can stem from certain situations. Trait anxiety, on the other hand, indicates long term or chronic anxiety as seen in persons with generalized anxiety.

Anxiety is not as prevalent as depression; nonetheless it affects millions of people's lives. We all know that exercise is a natural anti-depressant for the human body and mind. When dealing with panic attacks you must realize that there is something wrong physiologically and it's not just all in your head. So this program strengthens your nervous system to give you a healthier, more balanced physiologically sound human body. Meditation, quiet rest and relaxation techniques tend to help but there seems to be more physiological benefits in exercise programs.

Pharmacotherapy is treatment with medication. The most commonly used medications are tricyclic anti-depressants, high potency benzodiazepines, selective seretonin reuptake inhibitors (SSRIs) and monoamine oxidase inhibitors (MAOIs) (Hendrix, 1993; Paluska et al., 2000). It was discovered that panic attacks were diminished to null after following through with this 8-week program (to be explained in a later chapter). In the study by Paluska, et al. (2000) it is stated that "Anxiety symptoms and panic disorder also improve with regular exercise, and beneficial effects appear to equal meditation or relaxation." Even after a single session, physical activity has been linked to improved mood and creativity (Paluska et al., 2000). There is one thing that this program differs in however, and that is that you do not have to keep up continuous regular exercise after the 8th week of this program. No more exercise was needed to keep the panic attacks away. "Exercise seems to have similar efficacy to psychotherapy and provides no significant contraindications to the use of medications" (Paluska et al., 2000). In other words, it's safe to exercise while you're on medication and that exercise has similar effects to that of taking medication and/or receiving counseling. People with panic disorder tend to avoid exercise because they fear that it may be detrimental to their health and that it might even trigger an attack, when in fact, it is going to help reduce the symptoms (Paluska et al., 2000).

There are many people who have had panic attacks and have a lot of experience with them and have even been very successful in overcoming their problem. They may have attacks occasionally, but they're good at handling them and therefore do not allow the panic attacks to dominate their lives. This program seems to eliminate the attacks altogether. The fearful thoughts may arise but your body just doesn't seem to react in the same way physiologically. When trying to conduct studies about anxiety disorders, scientists use methods to induce panic. One such known method is by allowing the patient to breathe in more carbon dioxide. This will induce panic attacks. Another way is to have patients who are prone to having panic attacks injected with sodium lactate (the same chemical that builds up in the muscle during heavy exercise) (Hendrix, 1993). This will also induce panic attacks. Sodium lactate is also known as lactic acid. The lactic acid build up and the anaerobic exercise presented in this book is one connection to why this program helps to stop panic attacks. You will be performing anaerobic exercises (to be discussed), which helps your body handle lactic acid better. Here's how. When you lift an object or weight until you go to failure (can't go any further) you have gotten to that end point because of the build up of lactic acid in your muscles. This occurs because the body was unable to meet the high demands of energy and oxygen through the oxygenation process. (There's more on cell rate exchange in a later chapter). The anaerobic training over time causes your muscles and body to adapt to the lactic acid accumulation, therefore causing your threshold for panic attacks to be raised to a significantly higher level. The bottom line is that anxiety disorders, including panic disorder, seem to improve with regular physical exercise (Paluska et al., 2000). In addition to physical exercise, meditation and relaxation were highly effective in this program as well. The meditation is in prayer, the word of God and transforming your thought pattern to the thoughts in the Bible. The reason behind that is because Jesus Christ is the counselor in Isaiah 9:6, and in II Timothy 1:7: the Bible states, "For God has not given us the spirit of fear but of power, and of love, and of a sound mind." It's that simple. The breathing and relaxation technique is discussed in "The Breath of Life" chapter.

PART II
THE REMEDY

CHAPTER 7

Who is the Great Physician?

Have you ever seen a physician, or anybody for that matter, resurrect themselves back to life like Jesus Christ the Great Physician did for himself? If any physician knows about life and death, pain and sickness, this God-man Jesus Christ does.

In Isaiah 53:5 the Bible says "But he was wounded for our (the whole world's) transgressions, he was bruised for our iniquities; the chastisement of our peace was upon him; and with his stripes we are healed."

Then in I Peter 2:24 the Bible says, ". . . by whose stripes ye were healed." It was at the cross where Jesus Christ bore our (the entire world's) sins in his body on the tree (cross). Before he was crucified on the cross they dressed him in purple as a king and put a crown of thorns on his head to mock him. They whipped his back until stripes and welts swelled up and he bled. They even smote him in the face with the palms of their hands and nailed him to the cross to suffer. Although he was the Great Physician, they still continued to murder him. They mocked him further saying, "he saved others but himself he can not save." They were telling him that although he healed many and even raised people from the dead, he was not allowed to perform (not practice) his healing power (not an art) around them. Besides, they were insinuating that he was not legal by the law; because he didn't have a right to practice according to the religious leaders (especially on the Sabbath).

For all of those who have fears and anxieties, here is a session with the Great Physician that will move your soul to a more peaceful state.

In Mark 4:35 it reads, "And the same day, when the even was come, he saith unto them, Let us pass over unto the other side. And when they had sent away the multitude, they took him even as he was in the ship. And there were also with him other little ships. And there arose a great storm of wind, and the waves beat into the ship, so that it was now full. And he was in the hinder part of the ship, asleep on a pillow: and they awake him, and say unto him, Master, carest thou not that we perish? And he arose, and rebuked the wind, and said unto the sea, Peace, be still. And the wind ceased, and there was a great calm. And he said unto them, Why are ye so fearful? how is it that ye have not faith? And they feared exceedingly, and said to one another, What manner of man is this, that even the wind and the sea obey him?"

I was meditating one day when I took myself back to where I was at Jesus' feet in prayer and I remembered when he asked me personally, "why are ye so fearful?" I looked up at his face and honestly said, "Because I was scared to die" and he didn't flinch, waver or budge. He just looked at me with calmness, never loosing concentration. Just like he looked at those men in that boat when he asked them "Why are ye so fearful?"

He then said "peace be still" and there was a great calm. In my case, he didn't even say "peace be still" but I could feel it in my spirit because I knew that was what he'd say next. He was calm and no storm was upsetting him at all.

Even with me telling Him that I was scared to die, that didn't move Him at all. That's when I felt His spirit come into me and with me looking at Him the fear left. Now I understand it when he says in (II Tim. 1:7) "For God has not given us the spirit of fear; but of power, and of love and of a sound mind." I could then see plainly that the spirit of fear was upon me but now I have the spirit of love, and of power and a sound mind. The spirit of fear left. Now that that was all taken care of he asks the next question, "How is it that ye have no Faith?" I searched myself and I could not find any reason why I shouldn't have faith. But the more I beheld the Lord the more I could see that fear was keeping me from having strong faith. I know I have some faith because the word says He has dealt to everyman the measure of faith, but now with fear (and there is also doubt and unbelief that hinders as well) out of the way I was able to push all of my believing power or faith into his will. When I did this I no longer feared anything, not death, nor life, nor angels, nor anything.

I prayed this same prayer some time later and the Lord told me to "be of good cheer, I have overcome Death and Hell."

The Bible says in (I John 4:18) that ". . . perfect love casteth out fear because fear has torment . . ."

And then in Heb. 2:14-15 it talks about us being in bondage all our lifetime through fear of death because the devil had the power of death, but Jesus Christ destroyed the devil. And then he succoured me, just like he can succour you. He's the Great Physician that can calm any storm in anyone's life at any time. Now that's perfect peace.

CHAPTER 8

Praying For Answers

Listen, you will never know the power of prayer until you try it. People can't even explain how it works, but if God says it in his Holy Bible, then obey Him and do it. If he created the heavens and the earth and all that in them is, then he definitely knows how to handle some small time sore throat or any other seemingly difficult situation. Don't get discouraged when he doesn't answer immediately either. He's an on-time God. He's never too late and he's never too early, but you'll never know your prayer got answered without first asking the Lord for something through prayer. Philippians 4:6 says, "Be careful for nothing; but in everything by prayer and supplication with thanksgiving let your requests be made known unto God." Philippians 4:19 says, "But my God shall supply all your need according to his riches in glory by Christ Jesus." I knew quite a bit of this going through my ordeal while I was in those hospitals. I also had a tremendous headache that lasted for four years and no one could figure it out. I kept believing God was going to deliver me from all of this. I sometimes contemplate about when Joseph was sold by his brothers and later cast into prison. I just wonder about all of the thoughts and prayers that he thought and prayed while in prison. Then some forgetful, self-centered cupbearer forsook him and his promise to remind the king about Joseph interpretating his own dream. Thank God something caused him to remember. Then when the Pharaoh had a dream that no one could interpret, the cupbearer spoke up and said, "Hey, there's a man in prison who can interpret your dreams. He interpreted mine." Then God brought Joseph up out of the prison. The same way he brought me up and out. He was so wise because God was with him. He was found to be so wise that he was made ruler over all of Egypt. I believe Joseph was praying a lot while in that prison and it never left his mind that he needed to be delivered. And when he was delivered, God let him be the one that delivered the rest of his people (the Jews) during the great famine. The same that this book can do for you. If God can deliver me, then I now know how to deliver you. There's hard work ahead, but wisdom from God and his chosen people can tell you how to get delivered. When you have wisdom from God you have all knowledge and wisdom, period. The Bible says in Proverbs 21:30 "There is no wisdom nor understanding nor counsel against the Lord." Sometimes Lord I wonder, "How did I ever get into this mess?" So we sometimes ask "Why me?" People cry out "Why me, Lord?" and get angry at God as though he's picking on them. Sure your faith is being tried but he wants to see if anybody would search for his wisdom and knowledge as they search for riches of gold and silver. Read Deuteronomy 4:29: "But if from thence thou shalt seek the Lord thy God thou shalt find him if thou seek him with all thy heart and with all thy soul." Also in Jeremiah 29:13 it says, "And ye shall seek me, and find me when ye shall search for me with all your heart."

If you keep praying he'll show you how you can be someone special to him in his word. If you're sick, keep asking and he'll either perform a miracle instantaneously or give you a way to be healed over a process of time, even if it does take the use of medicine. I kept believing that he'd get me off of all medicine and he did.

Look at the woman which had an issue of blood again. She spent all her money and grew none the better, but rather was made worse.

Listen. If you want good things you need to pray and fast. You want to be healed? Pray and fast. That's how I learned how to get healed, body, mind, soul and spirit. Praying is how you make your personal appointment with the great physician Jesus Christ. And when he gives you an answer, well that's your very own prescription that he's prescribed to you. Prayer in the name of Jesus Christ is the answer, friend.

In Matthew 17:14-21, it reads: "And when they were come to the multitude, there came to him a certain man, kneeling down to him, and saying. Lord have mercy on my son: for he is a lunatick, and sore vexed: for oftimes he falleth into the fire, and oft into the water. And I brought him to thy disciples, and they could not cure him." Then Jesus answered and said, "O faithless and perverse generation, how long shall I suffer you? bring him hither to me." And Jesus rebuked the devil; and he departed out of him: and the child was cured from that very hour. Then came the disciples to Jesus apart, and said, "Why could not we cast him out?" And Jesus said unto them, "Because of your unbelief: for verily I say unto you, If ye have faith as a grain of mustard seed, ye shall say unto this mountain, Remove hence to yonder place: and it shall remove: and nothing shall be impossible unto you. Howbeit this kind goeth not out but by prayer and fasting." So we find that prayer and fasting helps your belief (faith).

The Bible also says in Mark 11:20-26: "And in the morning, as they passed by, they saw the fig tree dried up from the roots. And Peter calling to remembrance saith unto him, "Master, behold, the fig tree which thou cursedst is withered away." And Jesus answering saith unto them, "Have faith in God. For verily I say unto you, That whosoever shall say unto this mountain, Be thou removed, and be thou cast into the sea; and shall not doubt in his heart, but shall believe that those things which he saith shall come to pass; he shall have whatsoever he saith. Therefore I say unto you, what things soever ye desire, when ye pray, believe that ye receive them, and ye shall have them. And when ye stand praying, forgive, if ye have ought against any: that your Father also which is in heaven may forgive you your trespasses. But if ye do not forgive, neither will your Father which is in heaven forgive your trespasses."

So when you combine faith and forgiveness in your prayer, Jesus Christ says that ye shall have what things soever ye desire when you pray, if you will believe that you will receive them. He also said in John 15:7 that "If ye abide in me, and my words abide in you, ye shall ask what ye will, and it shall be done unto you." All things are possible to them that believe.

CHAPTER 9

Faith to Believe

When you pray, you really need to believe for it. If you don't believe for it, how in the world can it ever happen? People destroy themselves so bad with self-defeat by unbelief and doubting. Some are just ignorant and don't know any better, but others have no excuse at all. Now believe this or not, some people just like to be sick because they get so much attention for being sick. After so long they don't want to change from that. Now, I can't give you faith, but God has already given you faith. It says in Romans 12:3 "For I say, through the grace given unto me, to every man that is among you, not to think of himself more highly than he ought to think; but to think soberly, according as God hath dealt to every man the measure of faith." Hebrews 11:1 says, "Now faith is the substance of things hoped for, the evidence of things not seen." You can never stop someone's faith. Faith in God is the strongest power known to man. Faith can move mighty mountains. If there is an obstacle in your way, feed your faith the word of God. It says in Romans 10:17 "so then faith cometh by hearing and hearing by the word of God." Build it up. That's why the Lord put the ultimate hand book (Holy Bible) down here on Earth. He's the King of all kings and we are all in his kingdom or domain. He rules. Whether in heaven or earth, HE RULES. Besides, his kingdom is not of this world. It's a spiritual kingdom.

All this talk about a spiritual judgment and a spiritual Great Physician is not nonsense. Hebrews 11:3 says, "Through faith we understand that the worlds were framed by the word of God, so that things which are seen were not made of things which do appear." Hebrews 11:6 says, "But without faith it is impossible to please him; for he that cometh to God must believe that he is, and that he is a rewarder of them that diligently seek him." Through faith people were raised from the dead, withered hands were restored, lepers cleansed. Noah built an ark by faith by believing what the Lord said about the fact that it was going to rain and flood the whole earth. Hey, if these illnesses are floods that destroy, then truly this book is a rainbow to every sufferer of these syndromes. There's a promise (rainbow) in the sky and it's colorful. Every time you see one, God's talking. He's reminding us of his covenant with mankind. What do you think the blind man could look up and see? He couldn't see physically but he could see spiritually. There's now serious truth to the old saying, "Now I see says the blind man." But he didn't stay blind. God healed him, and it was manifested in his natural body. Sometimes in my prayers I'd ask the Lord "Why am I not getting healed? Would you heal me Lord, my heavenly Father? I'm asking you would you heal me in the name of Jesus Christ? I'm asking it in your name and I believe you for it." As I prayed and waited, I was determined to get an answer from the Lord. I was trying to be diligent. I pressed and pressed. And over time as I waited in silence he spoke to me. Remember those three words that I heard from God but didn't tell you what they were in Chapter 1? Well, here they are. He said "ONLY JUST BELIEVE." And I said to myself, "Lord is that you?" I cried and cried. Oh, master, thank you. Thank you God. In the name of Jesus Christ, I love you. At that time I was looking at a small wooden box with a picture of Jesus Christ on it and thought to myself, he spoke to me. "ONLY JUST BELIEVE." That's what he told me (but not audibly). It was deep in my heart and I could actually feel it. I searched the Bible to look where he said those precise words and the closest I could find was in Mark 5:36, ". . . Be not afraid, only believe." I knew this was the Lord. I meditated and meditated and said "Lord am I not believing?" But he didn't say that exactly. He said, "ONLY JUST BELIEVE." I told the Lord in all honesty "Little children do this all day long and I'm stumbling at the easiest part." Little children are so far ahead of me on this. But as I thought more, I remembered as a little child, I was sent to a church and I heard about this man that had a disease all over his body and was told by some special man that could hear from God that he was to go dip himself seven times into some river. I remember it so vividly. Later, as I learned more about the Bible, I found out it was Naaman who was sick and Elisha was the prophet which told Naaman what the Lord said for him to do in the Jordan River. And after he was healed Elisha wouldn't even take a gift (payoff) from Naaman.

So I kept thinking (meditating) and asked the Lord, would you increase my faith in the name of Jesus Christ? For the disciples asked the very same thing in the book of Luke. In Luke 17:5-10, it reads: "And the apostles said unto the Lord, Increase our faith. And the Lord said, If ye had faith as a grain of mustard seed, ye might say unto this sycamore tree, Be thou plucked up by the root, and be thou planted in the sea; and it should obey you. But which of you, having a servant plowing or feeding cattle, will say unto him by and by, when he is come from the field, Go and sit down to meat? And will not rather say unto him, Make ready wherewith I may sup, and gird thyself, and serve me, till I have eaten and drunken; and afterward thou shalt eat and drink? Doth he thank that servant because he did the things that were commanded him? I trow not. So likewise ye, when ye shall have done all those things which are commanded you, say, We are unprofitable servants: we have done that which was our duty to do." So when you say to yourself "It's my duty to do those things that you have commanded me to do." and really do them with the understanding that there is no special praise for what you've done, then your faith will be increased. In other words, we can never do enough for God because we will still be unprofitable servants. It's just our obligation.

So I spent time on learning how to believe and get unbelief out of the way. There's no room for doubt. If my faith could believe it, he was going to meet my faith with his power. "But how much could I believe him for?"

So after I really believed him, I went around telling my family and others that the Lord spoke to me and that he was going to heal me of this constant pain from FMS and MPS.

Consider Abraham, the Father of Faith, who staggered not at the promises of God, his belief was counted as Righteousness unto him (Romans 4:3). Romans 4:18-25 says that Abraham, "Who against hope believed in hope, that he might become the father of many nations, according to that which was spoken, *So shall thy seed be.* And being not weak in faith, he considered not his own body now dead, when he was about an hundred years old, neither yet the deadness of Sarah's womb: He staggered not at the promise of God through unbelief; but was strong in faith, giving glory to God; And being fully persuaded that, what he had promised, he was able also to perform. And therefore it was imputed to him for righteousness. Now it was not written for his sake alone, that it was imputed to him; But for us also, to whom it shall be imputed, if we believe on him that raised up Jesus our Lord from the dead; Who was delivered for our offences, and was raised again for our justification."

If you really want to be healed, you're going to have to have faith like that of faithful Abraham. "By faith Abraham, when he was called to go out into a place which he should after receive for an inheritance, obeyed; and he went out, not knowing whither he went" (Heb. 11:8). Like Abraham, you are being called to a place of Healing in your life. So won't you come and walk by faith like Abraham did?

I believe the Bible calls this touching the hem of God's garment. Just as the woman with an issue of blood did. For she said within her heart, "If I could but touch the hem of his garment I will be made whole." And sure enough after she pressed through the crowd she touched the hem of his garment and he looked around and asked, "Who touched me?" He felt virtue (POWER) leave him. Healing virtue. It went right into that woman and healed her issue of blood after twelve years of pain and suffering. He chose the poor of this world to be rich in faith. He looked at her and said, "Daughter, THY FAITH hath made thee whole." That's exercising spiritual understanding when we believe for God to do the things he said he came to do.

If you want to be healed, you must believe for it when you ask for it. You have to act on your faith because in James 2:26 it declares "For as the body without the spirit is dead, so faith without works is dead also." It's not enough to just believe, you have to act on that belief. Have faith and believe because if you doubt you will never get anything done. He opened my spiritual eyes so that I could see plainly. He opened my spiritual ears so that I could hear plainly. He healed my spiritual disease which was sin. He conquered death, hell and the grave and turned around and opened the door to eternal life for all. He says in John 10:9 "I am the door . . ." and in John 14:6 ". . . I am the way, the truth and the life: no man cometh to the Father, but by me." I believe him. I have faith he's going to raise me from the dead just like he delivered me from virtually all symptoms of these conditions. If you truly believe that God will heal you, you should get healed, just like the woman with the issue of blood did.

> ". . . If Thou canst believe, all things are possible to him that believeth."
>
> Mark 9:23

CHAPTER 10

What is the remedy?

There are a lot of discoveries and remedies known to man for various types of illnesses. And one of the most well known discoveries in the medical field was that of Alexander Fleming, who shared a Nobel Prize in 1945 for his medical discovery.

"Alexander Fleming (1881-1955) was a British bacteriologist who discovered penicillin" (Alexander Fleming, 2000).

Penicillin is a substance that's produced by mold, *Penicillin notatum* and is effective in killing many types of pathogenic bacteria without harming the cells of the human body.

In fact it was in 1928 that Fleming made this discovery and it was by accident. He was working on a bacteria called "*staphylococcus aureus* and had put aside some petri dishes that contained the cultures." Later he discovered that specks of green mold had appeared and killed the bacterial colonies around them. This effect was known as "antibiosis" (against life), and is where we derive the word anti-biotic (Alexander . . . , 2000).

Anti-biotic treatment is now widely used around the world.

Another accidental discovery (but not necessarily medical) was the discovery of Charles Goodyear (Charles Goodyear, 2001). He was born in New Haven, Connecticut on December 29, 1800. He accidentally dropped some rubber mixed with sulfur on a hot stove forming vulcanized rubber.

His discovery eventually came in use for many industrial companies for various purposes.

Rubber tires for automobiles and trucks are just some of the uses as a result of his accidental discovery. The Goodyear tire company still carries his name today (Charles . . . , 2001).

I've had a lot of hopes of overcoming these illnesses in the past. For instance, I used to hear how every cell in the body would renew itself every 7 yrs. I remember hoping for my 28th birthday for my cells to renew but I didn't get any better when they did, so that theory went down the tubes.

I've tried other books on chronic fatigue syndrome to no avail. I did their prescribed exercises, the prescribed medication protocol, the prescribed diet and still no results. I knew then that these people didn't know as much as they needed to. Besides, most didn't even have any of these syndromes to begin with.

The Lord says in Jeremiah 33:3 "Call unto me and I will answer thee and show thee great and mighty things which thou knowest not."

This is the exact procedure that I followed in order to get the results that I've gotten from this Remedy.

As time went by, I remember watching a program on body builders and coming to the realization that they have the strongest and healthiest muscles I've ever seen on the face of the earth.

That's another time I prayed and asked the Lord what I could do to strengthen up my back muscles. He let me know that I could weight lift to help build back the weak muscles. So I began to study and learn about proper weightlifting to just strengthen all of my muscles. I didn't know at the time that virtually all of my symptoms were going to disappear as a result of performing this program. That realization came some time later, like that of Alexander Fleming and Charles Goodyear.

And I still kept in my memory bank those three words from the Lord "ONLY JUST BELIEVE."

You may ask the question "What if I'm on medication?" Well that's alright too, as long as your doctor approves of you performing exercises.

So enough talk about the Remedy, right? You now want to know exactly what the Remedy is, right?

The remedy for FMS, MPS, CFS, GWS and Anxiety (Panic) Attacks is a combination of seeking God, diet, quality rest, exercise, herbal remedies and hot tub therapy combined to give ultimate results to patients.

So what we'll need to do for the body is maximize cellular respiration and increase metabolism while putting the highest quality of nutrients possible back into the cells without the use of medication (s).

This Remedy and the exercises in the following chapters help to flush out the cells at the best rate possible and remove the waste build up sites that form painful tender points and trigger points.

The natural remedy that worked

The natural remedy that worked is a combination of consuming CO-Q-10 with Ginkgo biloba as well as adding protein drinks to your diet, while performing aerobic and anaerobic exercises regularly. It is anaerobic exercise that rids the human body of tender points, trigger points, constant widespread musculoskeletal pain and Anxiety (Panic) attacks. And that is achieved without the use of any medication whatsoever.

CO-Q-10 really helps the body utilize oxygen for total respiratory improvement. It gives the heart more energy to help it work more efficiently. It also helps sustain the immune system. It is said that CO-Q-10 may help benefit trained athletes in performance and/or relief of chronic fatigue (Lee, 1987).

Ginkgo biloba will help open the capillaries to increase blood flow, especially to the brain. The capillaries in tender points and trigger points will also open more for better and increased cellular respiration. But keep the dosage at its minimum dosage.

A new study at the University of Alabama at Birmingham shows that FMS patients have diminished blood flow to parts of the brain and an increase in the chemical substance P which helps transmit pain signals (Researchers Find Abnormality in Fibromyalgia, 2001). Hence, pain amplification and Raynaud's phenomenon. Finally, there is some physical evidence to help suggest that the diagnosis of FMS is a real sickness.

So, getting proper blood flow restored to the muscles may help them relax better.

The protein mix drinks will allow cells to repair and regrow under the exercise regimen that's recommended. The amino acids may be used to help the brain produce proper amounts of chemicals, especially of the pain relieving type which will include endorphins. God's Remedy is the best natural remedy that really, really works. All patients may get health benefits from this program regardless of which of these syndrome(s) or conditions(s) they may have. In other words, this remedy is the same for FMS, MPS, CFS, CFIDS, GWS and Anxiety (Panic) Attacks.

LET'S REVIEW THE HYPOTHESIS

These exercises combined with a proper diet, supplements and hot tub therapy speed up cell rate exchange and actually help to push out excess waste from the sites of trigger points and tender points. The diet and supplements then replenish these sites with the most proper nutrition available.

Within the Earths' gravitational field, everything that goes up must come down. And so in a similar way every illness on Earth has a Remedy. Unfortunately, mankind has just not discovered all of them.

It would be in the best interest of the patients to use the recommended supplements for a perfect balance of nutrients since they are full of the proper nutrients (i.e., amino acids plus vitamins and minerals). It is believed that all of these combined is what is needed to get the cells working as close to normal as realistically possible. The anaerobic exercise burns out the stored energy (glycogen and others) and the hot tub therapy and exercises help to remove waste. Water is the ultimate lubricant to help wash the waste out of these cells, so be sure to drink lots of it. The gingko biloba and COQ_{10} help put more oxygen in the blood and in the cells. In this program we used efficiency and that is the most amount of help with the least amount of effort. By continuing this program over time, the build up sites (tender points and trigger points) will go down until they are completely gone because it repeatedly drains the cells and then replenishes them back again. This is great news for patients. This process can also help the brain regulate the body better since it will be receiving the necessary nutrients and amino acids which in turn will help the brain manufacture endorphins and other neurotransmitters more efficiently. Exercise alone can also help the brain regulate endorphins better. This hypothesis on removing waste sites (tender points and trigger points) by the repeated process of exercise, diet, hot tub therapy and rest will eventually win yourself the victory over this battle against your illness. Not only were primary trigger points alleviated but also associated trigger points disappeared with this program. No more need for painful massages with thumbs and elbows to relieve the trigger points and no more injections of corticosteroids or even stretch and spray are needed either.

The old theory was that gentle aerobic exercise was needed on a continuous basis. But this program does better than to require you to keep up that type of exercise on a continuous basis forever with no lasting results, because within 8 weeks you're done.

All of these herbal remedies combined give it a synergistic effect to give you ultimate benefits. It is the most efficacious program to date. This Remedy would have worked for people hundreds and even thousands of years ago had they known about it. When it comes to these illnesses the buck stops here. I'm not sending you around to the next person; we're fixing your illness here and now with this Remedy. God's Remedy is as solid as a rock. Even 100 years later this remedy will still be the same because it's as solid as a rock. If you're like everybody else, then you've prayed and prayed for an answer from God that you'd get healed somehow or someway. I believe your prayers have all been heard because this Remedy, "God's Remedy" is an answer to many prayers to restore your health back to normal.

CHAPTER 11

The Breath of Life

Genesis 2:7 says "And the Lord God formed man of the dust of the ground, and breathed into his nostrils the breath of life and man became a living soul." Now, Jesus Christ was made a quickening spirit. A spirit that can bring back to life something that was dead.

Read I Corinthians 15:45, "And so it is written, The first man Adam was made a living soul; the last Adam was made a quickening spirit."

Spiritually speaking we are all dead until we are born again as John 3:1-8 states. It declares that, "There was a man of the Pharisees, named Nicodemus, a ruler of the Jews: The same came to Jesus by night, and said unto him, Rabbi, we know that thou art a teacher come from God: for no man can do these miracles that thou doest, except God be with him. Jesus answered and said unto him, Verily, verily, I say unto thee, Except a man be born again, he cannot see the kingdom of God. Nicodemus saith unto him, How can a man be born when he is old? can he enter the second time into his mother's womb, and be born? Jesus answered, Verily, verily, I say unto thee, Except a man be born of water and of the Spirit, he cannot enter into the kingdom of God. That which is born of the flesh is flesh; and that which is born of the Spirit is spirit. Marvel not that I said unto thee, Ye must be born again. "The wind bloweth where it listeth, and thou hearest the sound thereof, but canst not tell whence it cometh, and whither it goeth: so is every one that is born of the spirit." When a person is born again they receive a second wind so to speak. An everlasting breath from God.

Now I did this for my spiritual life, but as far as for our physical or natural breath here on earth, we normally would not need instructions on how to breathe unless we became ill.

You can live for about a month without food and maybe a week without water, but you will die in a matter of minutes without air (oxygen). Not enough emphasis has been placed on breathing. So I hope to encourage you enough so that you will try breathing exercises of which could benefit you greatly.

In respiration, all cells must have a continuous supply of oxygen and must continuously eliminate carbon dioxide (CO_2) as a waste product (World Book,

1977). Please understand that food is loaded with carbon dioxide and breathing combines oxygen with water and food giving off carbon dioxide, heat and energy as a by product.

There are three types of respiration: external, internal and cellular (World Book, 1977). External respiration is when you breathe in oxygen and it mixes with your blood through the lungs (World Book, 1977). So just being outside and breathing in fresher open air would help you in this way. Once outside, you are in contact with fresher air that has a plenteous supply of fresh oxygen (about 21% of the atmosphere), instead of being indoors with just stale, recycled air. Being outside makes people really want to "breathe in" so much deeper too. Try it and you'll be able to tell the difference. External respiration is the only form of respiration you really have physical control over. I'm not referring to diet and exercise. I hope this program covers that very well. If you diet right, exercise right, and breathe right (deeper), your body can't help but to become as efficient and healthy as God will let it.

Internal respiration is your blood carrying oxygen to all cells and carrying carbon dioxide away from all cells (World Book, 1977). Cellular respiration is when oxygen is burned within the cells with various nutrients to give the cell energy and give off CO_2 as a waste (World Book, 1977). Living cells have respiratory enzymes that cause respiration to occur in the cells. That is, the respiratory enzymes act on the oxygen and nutrients through an extremely intricate process to produce carbon dioxide, heat and energy (World Book, 1977). We can only help our external respiration through physical breathing exercises. We can help internal and cellular respiration by taking certain helpful remedies and even by consuming small amounts of apple cider vinegar. This helps to oxygenate your blood.

CO-Q-10 also helps internal and cellular respiration because it helps the body utilize oxygen better. Ginkgo biloba helps this as well by dilating blood vessels and allowing better blood flow to the body (especially capillaries).

Efficiency Diagram
Water + Food + Oxygen = Carbon Dioxide + Energy (heat)

If oxygen levels aren't high enough you will not be able to produce proper amounts of energy or efficiently dispose of waste (carbon dioxide) (World Book, 1977). Your body becomes less energetic and less efficient, and healing will take longer.

So in order to make respiration more efficient, you must learn to breathe deeper than what you have been doing.

After practicing breathing you might be thinking about breathing deeper on a more frequent basis, but in time it will become natural to you and you won't even have to consciously think about it so much. So once you're back into shape it's easier to stay there. It's getting back into shape that requires so much proper attention.

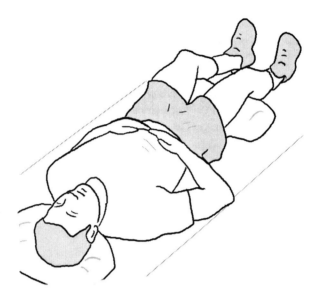

Figure 11-1: Breathing Exercise.

Let's begin. Lie down on a bed with a pillow under your head (not too high, but level) (See Figure 11-1) and place a pillow under your knees as well. Close your eyes and pretend you are looking at the tip of your nose. Looking down like this gives you better concentration. Now place your hands softly on your stomach below your navel and breathe right into your own hands. Feel your stomach rise up smoothly and go down smoothly. As you focus, concentrate on being relaxed. Don't force your breathing too hard; instead, let air come in your nose and go out of your mouth as relaxed as possible. Especially for panic attacks, this same breathing technique (slowly into your nose and out of your mouth) can help to prevent hyperventilation (a pattern of short breaths that can trigger or exacerbate panic attacks). Let your lungs feel the relaxed stretch. Focus on your lungs expanding wider and wider in a relaxed state, but don't force it. After you've done fifteen breaths, move your hands up onto the lowest end of your rib cage. Now focus on feeling the breathing into your hands into your midsection. You should feel the midsection rising and expanding outward. After fifteen breaths move your hands to your upper chest. Focus on feeling the lungs expand in your upper chest. Perform fifteen breaths. Next, slowly breathe into your upper chest and keep breathing until your midsection expands. Keep breathing evenly until your stomach is fully expanded. Then slowly let all of the air out and feel your lungs and chest relax and sink deep down. Perform fifteen of these and relax.

Most people use their hands on their stomach, but you can try using a folded towel on the lower part of your stomach while you're breathing. It may help you visualize what you're doing much more easily.

If you want to start out easier you may perform five breaths for the lower stomach, five breaths for the midsection, five breaths for the upper section and five breaths for complete breathing exercises. Complete breathing is causing all three areas to fill as you inhale before beginning to exhale. Do this every day.

You may start at the upper chest and work down if you'd like. If you get good and enjoy it, you may perform it as long or as frequently as you'd like. Although I recommend not going over forty-five minutes per session unless you are otherwise inclined to do so. If you get a headache, it is an indication you are straining too hard. This is supposed to be relaxing. Keep your jaw relaxed and also the muscles in your face, head and neck. Focus on the muscles allowing you to breathe to become strong and graceful. Some martial artists really know how to breathe this way and even do it standing up. They use this same breathing technique to help them focus and to gather strength. The Japanese call their stomach area the "Hara."

Whenever you need to lay down during the day due to fatigue you may want to use this technique to keep a generous supply of oxygen going into your body for more energy. Just lie down on your bed for about 5 to 10 minutes as often as you need to. Lie there until you stretch your arms and legs out completely and maybe lie there until you yawn. Then perform these breathing exercises. This technique used frequently really helps you feel refreshed for the next few hours until you may want to do it again. Keep in mind; you're not going to have to always do this after you've successfully completed this program. This energy is not like a drug in which the effects are over intense. In reality you may not feel much energy at all, but on a cellular level you know you are steadily making progress. We must be as efficient as we can become in order to feel substantial improvement. With any one of these illnesses, it takes endurance. You may want to practice breathing for a whole week or two before you start exercising (to be discussed). This will get your body used to utilizing oxygen more efficiently because it eases stress. Another benefit of breathing is that it can actually help you lose weight by helping to burn off more fuel without exercising. This is especially good if you are overweight with these illnesses. When you start to exercise and it sets you back too far, then you have pushed too hard too soon.

Once you find the right pace then you've got it made because you'll be able to increase your physical stamina, get out of pain and get relief from virtually all symptoms.

So you must first start breathing, then add aerobic exercise to that, and then finally of course anaerobic exercise. Once you're out of pain and have no more tender points or trigger points then you can discontinue the anaerobic exercises. You may want to continue some aerobic exercise because it will keep you in shape and help give you energy. But if you must stop aerobic exercising, by all means keep the breathing exercises going. You may use breathing as an exercise even when you're disabled or have grown to an old age.

During normal breathing we only breathe in and out about one-seventh of the air in our lungs (World Book, 1977). The new air then mixes with the old. If a person is breathing quietly they may inhale about one pint of air per breath. That's what is known as tidal air. That's enough air to carry out normal body functions. On the other hand a person who is exercising can inhale about one gallon of air. This is called vital capacity (World Book, 1977). From one pint to one gallon is quite a difference. So during these breathing exercises you are trying to get your lungs to stretch out as if you were exercising strenuously, but yet relaxed. Then when you do start exercising it won't be such a shock to your system and you will be able to recover from each workout easier during training.

Most exercise programs start you right off with the physical exercises and then let your lungs recover afterwards. But with an illness like FMS, MPS, CFS, GWS or AA your game plan has to be strategically better prepared. It's hard enough just coping with getting around from day to day when you start exercising, so you can only imagine how much breathing will benefit and help you recuperate each day from strenuous exercises. If you have FMS, MPS, CFS, GWS or AA, I have a hunch you probably haven't been exercising or breathing as deeply as you should. So today is a good day to start. Furthermore, these exercises could also help with the breathing abnormalities that go with these illnesses. They may not correct this problem altogether but with the aerobic and anaerobic exercises combined, it should. If you sprint a few times during your aerobic training on a treadmill or cycle (to be discussed), it should help to totally correct the unsynchronized breathing problem. There is more on that in "The Proper Regimen" chapter.

Chapter 12

The Proper Diet

Let's talk about diet. To understand diet better, we must understand that the energy value of food is counted in calories, and so is the energy that is burned during daily activities.

Calorie is the unit of measurement used to measure heat in the metric system. Let's look at an example. Suppose you have one thousand grams of water and you wanted to raise its temperature by one degree Celsius, it would require one calorie of heat to do so. So when you perform activities your body burns calories. When we were very young most of us were very active and we burned a lot of calories very quickly. We also ate lots of food (especially sugary foods), which put calories into our bodies to be burned. So when we were highly active our bodies heated up significantly while we were running and playing. Unfortunately, now that we are older, we no longer run around like we used to nor do we heat our bodies up for long periods of time anymore in order to burn off so many calories. Therefore our metabolism becomes less efficient in burning off fuel (calories). Trying to get back to where we heat our bodies up to burn more calories by activity is where the body has the strongest potential to heal itself.

This would include using up the stored energy (glycogen and fat) in cells by activity. Then once the energy is burned it becomes a waste product (carbon dioxide). The waste product is then washed out by the water that we drink, so always drink plenty of water during any exercise program. Now that your cells are being used more you must also eat the proper diet that will replenish the cells with fresh nutrients (vitamins, minerals, proteins, fats, and carbohydrates). This will not only revitalize your energy supply but will also help to repair and correct any illness or injury the body may have more efficiently. For example, a sprained wrist can heal over time without any bodily exercise, but it will heal faster if that person is in fit condition from exercise. He can actually keep the exchange rate of new fuel (proper food) into the cells up at a faster more efficient rate, even while at rest. This would allow new growth and repair to happen at a faster rate. Thus, the more fit a person is, the faster he can recover from injury or illness. So when someone has FMS or any of these other conditions they may no longer want to exercise because of the pain and fatigue. They are tired and hurting. Most patients try to do as little as possible and this slows down the rate of metabolism. Some do as little as possible in fear that their condition will be aggravated or even get worse. This prevents and slows down cell growth and repair. While it is not fully understood what is causing FMS, MPS, CFS, CFIDS, GWS or AA (there are only theories and only treatments), I know from first hand experience that this program based on these known principles have helped me to get great healing. It brought my metabolism up, helped to give me more strength and energy, helped to regain my concentration and the most desired of all, helped to stop the constant pain, the tender points, and trigger points. It is still unknown in exact medical terms how this program works to achieve these results, but we just know that it does and it has given the greatest desired results (without the use of medications) than any other treatment plan thus far.

Most of the time, you don't always need to know how something works in order for it to benefit you. For example, when you use a key to open your car door and then to start the engine you may not need to know every intricate detail about how it works, but you just have faith and trust that it will, and of course it does. That's the same for this program.

By the way, the PDR (Physician's Desk Reference) is full of medications of which scientists and physicians do not know exactly how they work. They cannot explain it in exact medical terms, but they just know that by using certain types of medicines they can achieve the desired results. And that's what counts, "desired results."

When the word diet is mentioned, most people associate it with starvation. But when following this program you will be glad to know that there are no crash diets nor is there room for eating a lot of junk food. When a person exercises frequently their need for proper nutrition is increased. By the way, you will not have to skip meals either. Growing and repairing muscles and nerves need proper nutrition and healthy eating is the way it should be done. Don't become too alarmed, you will not work out long enough in this program to even worry about having huge muscles like those in body building competitions. But to get healthier I believe you will need to grow and tone a little bit of muscle to ensure deep healing. When your diet and exercise is proper, you will add and tone muscle while losing fat with no starvation. With this program your body will receive the proper balance of protein, carbohydrates and fats.

Protein

Protein is absolutely essential for the structure and function of all cells (Kennedy and Greenwood-Robinson, 1987). That goes for the growth, repair and maintenance for virtually all body tissues. Bones, muscles, skin and other solid body parts are mostly made up of proteins. Proteins are a necessity for living things to live. Proteins are what repair damaged cells and also build new tissues. We get protein from meat, fish, poultry, eggs (especially egg whites), dairy products, grains (cereals) and vegetables. If you've ever heard people refer to the Bible concerning themselves being a vegetarian, according to Genesis 1:29 in the Old Testament, then you will have to also understand that today we are not under the old dispensation but under the new dispensation. And that means we're living in the New Testament era. I Timothy 4:1-5 in the new testament says, "Now the Spirit speaketh expressly, that in the latter times some shall depart from the faith, giving heed to seducing spirits, and doctrines of devils; Speaking lies in hypocrisy; having their conscience seared with a hot iron; Forbidding to marry, and commanding to abstain from meats, which God hath created to be received with thanksgiving of them which believe and know the truth. For every creature of God is good, and nothing to be refused, if it be received with thanksgiving: For it is sanctified by the word of God and prayer." But if you're a vegetarian then that will still be alright too. The old theory that eating excessive protein will help your muscles grow faster is not necessarily a true one either. It is now understood that the excessive protein that is not used by your body is stored away as fat (Kennedy . . . , 1987). The truth of the matter is that the body uses very little protein for energy as long as there are plenty of carbohydrates and fats available to be burned (Kennedy . . . , 1987).

Here's what happens while digesting food. The foods are broken down into amino acids (Kennedy . . . , 1987). These amino acids are the building blocks of proteins and are also what the body uses in order to manufacture proteins. They are used for maintenance, repair, and new cell growth for all cells in the body (Kennedy . . . , 1987). There are twenty-two amino acids and ten of them must be supplied by the food that we eat because our bodies don't manufacture them, therefore making them essential. Soy protein provides all twenty-two amino acids. Soy protein is also safe for diabetics and hypoglycemics.

In conjunction with aerobic and anaerobic training (weight lifting) you will need to use a protein mix supplement.

The best protein mix on the market for this program is American Whey™ made by American Sports Nutrition™. American Whey™ has been voted the best tasting protein mix on the market by their distributors. American Whey™ is 100% natural with no harmful artificial sweeteners, colors or preservatives. It has natural flavors and a natural sweetener. There's no ginseng, bee pollen, creatine, xenadrine, ephedrine, ma huang or caffeine added.

The American Whey™ protein mix is very easily dissolved for the body's maximum abortion. Just stir or shake, no blender is needed. This saves time, money and energy.

You may want to find you a quality shaker for your drinks because it really makes mixing your drinks a breeze.

American Whey™ protein mix has 104 calories per serving. Less than 1 gram of fat. 0 mg of cholesterol. Trace amounts of sodium with no added sodium. 6 grams of carbohydrates and 20 grams of protein. That's 0 grams of sugar per serving. It has a very small amount of sugar, less than 1 gram per serving and it is in the form of crystallized fructose (fruit sugar). It's also low in iron. It's even lactose free. It's sweetened with stevia, not phenylalanine; and doesn't contain stimulants that can be harmful to your nervous system. Stevia is a safe and natural sweetener that grows naturally, mostly in South America. It's safe, especially compared to saccharin or phenylalanine products.

You'll be needing about 2 ½ to 3 servings per day.

½ of a serving 1 hour before work out, 1 serving after workouts and one at bedtime. You'll still need to meet the recommended daily amounts of carbohydrates in order to restore glycogen levels after workouts. This is very important, so be sure to watch your diet for that.

You may mix your protein mix with whole milk, 2% milk, 1% milk, skim milk, milk substitute, your favorite juice or even water.

The "American Whey" protein mix comes in seven delicious flavors: creamy vanilla, double chocolate, wild berry, tropical banana, orange creamsicle, peach cobbler and natural.

Use the mix for the first 2-4 weeks while you are getting ready to perform anaerobic exercises as outlined in stage VII (the final stage of the program) of chapter 14 "The Proper Regimen." Once you're in stage VII consume about 2½ to 3 servings of protein mix per day for about 8 weeks or until you are completely finished with the program.

Even on rest days, be sure to take your protein mix. Do not use "American Whey" as your sole source of nutrition. Eat your ordinary meals along with it or use in between meals. If you begin to gain weight, cut back just ½ serving per day of the mix. If you still continue to gain weight then you might consider cutting back just ½ serving more per day. Any time you start an exercise program, your body will automatically gain a little weight, but over a short period of time it will lose that small portion of weight and probably even more. So, give it time to see if the immediate weight gain will taper back down before discontinuing any servings because your body desperately needs the nutrition during the program. Once you're finished with the program you may continue any leftover mix at about 1 serving per day for maintenance. You will also need to take additional supplements.

Country Life® vitamins have been around for over 25 years and have some of the best products on the market. They even have a GMP seal of approval by the National Nutritional Foods Association (NNFA). The NNFA has started the Good Manufacturing Practices (GMP) program to help regulate the manufacturing of dietary supplements. Country Life® currently exceeds their guidelines, which is one of the reasons they have the (GMP) seal of Approval. There are very few companies that meet or exceed this GMP approval and Country Life® is one of them.

As a part of this program you will also need to take an all-around multiple vitamin. The best hypo-allergenic all around multiple vitamin for this program is Daily Total One Rapid Release tablets by Country Life®.

Country Life® Daily total one Rapid Release tablets are tolerated well by even the most highly allergic individuals. They contain no yeast, wheat, gluten, milk, salt, sugar, starch, preservatives or artificial colors.

Here's what they contain:

Vitamin A with 50% as Beta Carotene	Vitamin C
Vitamin D	Vitamin E
Thiamin (B-1)	Riboflavin (B-2)
Niacin	Vitamin B-6
Folic Acid	Vitamin B-12
d-Biotin	pantothenic Acid
Calcium	Iron
Iodine	Magnesium
Zinc	Selenium
Manganese	Chromium
Potassium	choline Bitartrate
Inositol	Betaine HCL
PABA	Lemon Bioflavonoids
Rutin	

Be sure to take one a day after a meal, preferably 1 hour before workouts. But anytime will be alright as long as you'll be taking one every day.

Country Life® Daily Total One's also come in Iron free Daily Total One's in case you can't have the iron. They contain the same exact ingredients except for no iron. You'll also need to take Country Life® C_0Q_{10} and Ginkgo Biloba every day.

Country Life® Coenzyme Q_{10} 100mg caps contain no yeast, corn, wheat, soy, gluten, milk, salt, sugar, starch, preservatives or artificial colors.

Country Life® Ginkgo Biloba extract caps have 60mg of Ginkgo Biloba extract per capsule. It contains no yeast, corn, wheat, gluten, milk, salt, sugar, starch, preservatives or artificial colors.

Country Life® has the best products for this program.

I've laid out two basic kits for this program. The first is a basic complete supply kit and the second is a basic maintenance kit. You will have every supplement that you're going to need to finish this program when you order these products to make your own kit. Both kits should be fairly safe for diabetics and non-diabetics. Diabetics are advised to consult with their physician before using any supplement, diet or exercise program.

The basic complete supply kit contains C_0Q_{10}, Ginkgo Biloba, an all around multiple vitamin, and sugar free protein mix. The American Whey™ doesn't contain high amounts of carbohydrates nor excess sugar like other mixes, but still provides excellent nutrition for protein. It's designed to keep sugars and carbohydrates low but protein high in order to be beneficial and safe.

The maintenance supply kit contains: C_0Q_{10}, an all around multiple vitamin, and sugar free protein mix. The maintenance supply kit is designed to keep you at your best and is not mandatory for keeping symptoms away. But it will make you feel more energetic without the use of harmful stimulants. The Ginkgo Biloba was not required either, but may help fibrofog if that is a lingering symptom for you after you've been through the entire program.

The complete supply kit will contain enough protein mix to finish the entire program. That's about 3 servings per day of the protein mix for about 120 days (133 days to be more exact), 120 days supply of the C_0Q_{10}, Ginkgo Biloba, and an all around multiple vitamin.

If you think you can't afford this program, you might ask your church or other support group to help you get it. You really need your healing and I want to hear of you making a solid recovery. I want to hear about your miracle of healing. The Remedy is outlined in this book making it all very simple for you.

There are actually (2) kits to chose from.

Kit #1   4 month complete supply kit

133 day 25lbs. American Whey™ (about 3 per day)

2 x 60 day supply of C_0Q_{10} 100mg. Country Life® (1 per day)

2 x 60 day supply of Ginkgo Biloba Country Life® (1 per day)

2 x 60 day supply of Daily Total One Rapid Release with or without Iron all around multiple vitamin Country Life® (1 per day)

and

Kit #2   4 month maintenance kit

160 day 10lbs. Bucket of American Whey™ (about 1 per day)

2 x 60 day supply of CoQ10 100mg. Country Life® (1 per day)

2 x 60 day supply of Daily Total One Rapid Release with or without Iron all around multiple vitamin Country Life® (1 per day)

Order the appropriate amounts of supplements according to the kit you need. These companies will deliver to any destination in the world.

For American Whey™ protein mix call American Sports Nutrition™ at:

1(888) 462-5671 Toll Free and
1(203) 639-8189 International
(See Appendix A and C)

For Country Life® C_0Q_{10}, Ginkgo Biloba and an all around multiple vitamin (Daily Total One Rapid Release caps) call VNF Nutrition at:

1(800) 681-7099 Toll Free and
1(631) 689-6433 International
(See Appendix A and C for VNF Nutrition and Country Life® vitamins)

If you order through the 800# you'll get these products at a discount price. So go to the phone, order the products and start your program now.

The protein mix contains the following eighteen amino acids:

L-Alanine	L-Glycine	L-Proline
* L-Arginine	* L-Histidine	L-Serine
* L-Isoleucine	* L-Threonine	L-Aspartic Acid
* L-Leucine	* L-Tryptophan	L-Tyrosine
L-Cystine	* L-Lysine	* L-Valine
L-Glutamic Acid	* L-Phenylalanine	* L-Methionine

• = Ten essential amino acids

Figure 12-1: Amino Acids.

I fully believe that drinking these protein drinks which already have amino acids ready for absorption was vitally important in restoring my muscles, nerves and connective tissues back to as close to normal as possible. The protein mix and supplements give you most of the energy you will need for this program. Without the protein mix and supplements you'll never have the proper nutrition to carry out this program due to all of the exercises required. If you try without it, you will only further the fatigue that you're already experiencing. Just taking the regimen of the multi-vitamin, protein mix, ginkgo biloba and C_0Q_{10} will help you feel so much better too. So even if you don't want to go through the physical exercise regimen you can still take the best combination of supplements to get some health benefits. It's better than taking nothing. Remember, all of this extra protein, if not used, is stored away as fat. Too much carbohydrates and fats will be stored as body fat as well. So be sure you don't consume too much.

Carbohydrates

Carbohydrates are fruits, vegetables, grains, breads and sweet sugary foods to give the body more energy (Kennedy . . . , 1987). You will need a lot of carbohydrates because that will be your source of energy when you go to perform your exercise routines. In short, Carbohydrates keep energy levels up.

After realizing you will be able to eat some sugary foods for energy, this diet doesn't sound so bad after all, does it? But again, use moderation when eating sweets.

When carbohydrates are digested they are broken down into glucose which is blood sugar. This glucose is used for energy by your central nervous system and red blood cells. If your body does not use the glucose quickly, it will be stored in the liver and muscles as glycogen. Glycogen is where your energy comes from when you are performing your exercise. You will deplete most glycogen during a strenuous work out. So replenishing your body with the proper diet will restore these levels again (Kennedy . . . , 1987).

The sugar intolerance seems to be so much better with this program and yes, milk does seem to help keep sugar levels closer to their normal levels (Williamson, 1996).

Once again if you're a diabetic you must follow your doctor's instructions for your diet.

If you don't eat enough carbohydrates daily you will be tired and sluggish when it's time to exercise. Doing that will defeat the entire purpose of this program. If you have FMS, or any of these conditions, you are probably already tired and fatigued. So be sure to eat plenty of carbs so that when you exercise you will not cause your body to have fatigue amplified to such an extreme that you will only end up in a bed for days or weeks to recover. Speaking from experience, when you start exercising you will need to rest more to recuperate. Sometimes I felt so tired that I wanted to give up, but I knew I needed to strengthen myself. Plus, I'd remember that old cliche "The more you exercise, the more you can exercise." This makes sense once you understand the metabolism of the cells burning calories, washing out the waste and replenishing the cells back with proper nutrients, and then starting the cycle all over again.

There are two categories of carbohydrates: simple and complex. Simple carbohydrates are broken down within minutes of consumption and bring your glucose levels up quickly (Kennedy . . . , 1987). In return your pancreas responds by producing a surge of insulin which will rapidly bring your glucose level back down. And when this happens you will not feel so energetic, but rather weak, sluggish and even shaky (Kennedy . . . , 1987).

On the other hand, complex carbohydrates will supply a steady and constant supply of energy because your body breaks these down more slowly. So you'll be better off consuming plenty of complex carbohydrates instead of simple carbohydrates. Pasta is a good source of complex carbohydrates. The calories you get from carbohydrates should be from about 50% to 60% of your complete dietary intake.

Eating lots of fresh fruits and vegetables instead of lots of meat and dairy products really helps to keep the negative cognitive problems into remission. The memory of most patients with these illnesses seem to be stuck in a mode where they can't handle the stress load of higher functioning capabilities all day long, compared to those who do not have them.

Fats

Fats must be included in your diet in order to stay healthy. Fats are what supply the body with fatty acids for chemical activities like growth, metabolism and the manufacturing of sex hormones and cell membranes (Kennedy . . . , 1987). We need fat to help absorb vitamins A, D, E, and K (Kennedy . . . , 1987). It also helps to absorb calcium. Fat supplies nine calories of energy per gram. That's more than twice as much as protein or carbohydrates. Besides adding flavor and aroma, fats satisfy the feeling of hunger and they are also a very important source of energy for basal metabolism (Foods That Harm, Foods That Heal, 1997).

There are drawbacks, however, to a high fat diet. It can lead to obesity, cause elevated cholesterol levels, increase risk of heart disease, circulatory disorders, strokes and even cancer (Kennedy . . . , 1987). So please don't go overboard just because fats are supposed to keep you healthy. Only about 25%-30% of your calories should consist of fats (Kennedy . . . , 1987). And there are different kinds of fats as well.

There are saturated fats which are found in butter, hard cheese, palm and coconut oils (Foods . . . , 1997). Also fatty meats have a high percentage rate of saturated fats.

There are mono-unsaturated fatty acids which are found in olive oil, canola oil and foods like avocados, nuts and seeds (Foods . . . , 1997). Remember olive oil, canola oil and certain nuts contain polyunsaturated fats which are important.

There are polyunsaturated fats as well, which are; corn, other vegetable oils, fish oils and oily fish (Foods . . . , 1997). These also contain two types of essential fatty acids, omega 6 and omega 3. Omega 6, which is derived from linoleic acid, can be obtained through corn, safflower, soybean, and sunflower oils. Omega 3, which is derived from linolenic acid, comes from grapeseed and evening primrose oils, walnuts and oily fish like mackerel, sardines and salmon. Transfatty acids are hydrogenated oils such as margarine and processed foods such as pies, cakes, chips and such (Foods . . . , 1997). However, these are not the most favorable sources of fats.

Most of the fats are good for you except transfatty acids and you may also want to consider cutting back on the saturated fats (Foods . . . , 1997). Always remember to keep fats in moderation.

Here's how to figure your diet:

50%-60% of calories from carbohydrates
Less than 30% of calories from fat
20%-25% of calories from protein

Let's say you eat a bowl of raisin bran cereal with 2% milk, toast and jelly with a glass of orange juice. Use a chart like this to work from:

FOOD	AMOUNT	FAT	CARB.	PROTEIN
Cereal	1 cup	1.5 gm	47 gm	6 gm
Milk	1 cup	5 gm	12 gm	8 gm
Toast	2 slices	1.5 gm	25 gm	4 gm
Jelly	1 tbsp.	0	14 gm	0
Orange Juice	8 oz.	0	26 gm	2 gm
Total		8 gm	124 gm	20 gm

Figure 12-2: Food Values.

Calories per gram:

Fat 9   Carbohydrate 4   Protein 4

Let's look at just the cereal.

You take the fat grams from the cereal (1.5) and multiply it by 9 (fat calories) which is 1.5 x 9 = 13.5 fat calories.

Next take the carbohydrate grams (47) and multiply it by 4 (carbohydrate calories) which is 47 x 4 = 188 calories from carbohydrates.

The next step is to multiply the protein grams (6) by calories per gram of protein (4) which gives you 6 x 4 = 24, the total calories of protein is 24.

Add the carb calories with the fat calories and protein calories to get your total.

188 + 13.5 + 24 = 225.5 calories. The total calories are 225.5 for just the bowl of cereal not including the milk.

To find the percentage of protein, fats, and carbs, simply divide the 225.5 total calories into the total calories of proteins (24) and you should get about 10.6% of calories from protein, 83.4% for carbs and 5.9% for fats. Then to figure the entire breakfast:

	FAT	CARB	PROTEIN
Total	8 gm	124 gm	20 gm

Convert the grams into calories like this:

8 gm fat x 9 cal per fat gm = 72 fat calories

124 gm carbs x 4 cal per carb = 496 carb calories

20 gm protein x 4 cal per protein gm = 80 protein calories

This gives us 648 total calories. Divide the 648 calories into the protein calories (80), the carbohydrate calories (496) and the fat calories (72) to get the percentage of each:

Protein is	11.1%
Carbohydrates is	76.5%
Fats is:	12.3%

You will need to increase the protein for the next few meals and lower the carbs just a little. The fat is slightly low but could still be within normal range considering you still have two or three meals left to eat. Remember to add in your protein mix as well. You don't have to be exact but just keep your diet as close to this as reasonably possible. This diet may seem difficult, but it's not that hard after all.

Protein requirements drop gradually over a period of time as we get older. If you are a woman age 25 and weigh 150 pounds you will need about 50 grams or so of protein. If you gain weight because you are eating too much protein, fats and carbs, then cut back because your requirement is a lot less than what you're eating. There is no true set formula for how much protein every person in the world needs at this time, only recommendations. Our metabolism changes even within our own bodies constantly, therefore changing the food requirements as they are needed to meet the demands on the body.

Additional Diet Tips

Here are some additional diet tips to remember for a proper diet:

- Cut down on caffeine
- Avoid alcohol
- Eat salty foods using moderation if blood pressure is low (a common finding in FMS patients)
- Avoid neurotoxins like phenylalanine which tend to swell and destroy nerves and induce pain

After completing this program and being relieved of so many symptoms, I resumed eating anything I wanted and neither the constant muscle pains, trigger points nor tender points have come back on me. But you must eat well during this program. Do what you want to once you're out of pain but while training you must abide by the complete diet and exercise regimen. It's only sensible because this is what works.

You will get all of the vitamins and minerals you'll need from your all around daily multiple vitamin caps. You may discontinue the mix when you have completed this program, or you may choose to stay on the maintenance plan. To stay on the maintenance plan, just cut the protein mix servings down to 1 per day and continue taking the all around multiple vitamin, and the C_0Q_{10}. The Ginkgo biloba may be discontinued if you prefer.

BMR

Knowing about the BMR (basal metabolic rate) is something that can really help you. The BMR is the number of calories required to maintain your present weight day after day (Kennedy . . . , 1987). One way to guess at it is to multiply your current weight by ten. Let's say 150 pounds is your weight then you would need approximately 1500 calories to support your current weight. Of course, you must figure in any exercise you do. Then if you used 300 calories in exercise you would need 1800 calories to maintain your current weight. Do not try to lose weight quickly by dropping off the number of calories you consume too fast. This diet is to get you as healthy as you can get. You'll lose weight by increasing exercise or decreasing caloric intake or a combination of both. If you slow the caloric intake down too much, your basal metabolism rate may make a self-adjustment to a slower rate and you will be tearing down the objective of this program. Lose weight slowly and over a period of time, not all at once (Kennedy . . . , 1987). This diet is for helping with FMS and the other conditions. It is not a quick weight loss program. It is meant to stimulate a slight growth in your muscles, not a sharp decrease in fat.

When you exercise, use a chart similar to the one shown below which shows you how many calories you can burn in one hour of the exercise of your choice.

ACTIVITY	CALORIES BURNED/HR
Cycling—Moderate	250
Cycling—Fast	400-650
Weight Lifting	300-500
Cross Country Skiing	700
Jogging	700-950
Jumping Rope	750
Running	900
Swimming	250-500
Walking—Slow	210
Walking—Moderate	325
Walking—Fast	450
(Various sources)	

Figure 12-3: Calorie Burning chart.

Figuring in your exercise with your calories will help you locate your BMR more accurately. Eat some salty foods to help your hypotension if you have it, but by all means avoid excessive salt. Sports drinks are okay as long as you consume small quantities because consuming too much will make you feel weak and tired (worse than before you drank it). Moderation in all things is the key.

Water

Water is the most important nutrient of all (Kenney . . . , 1987). It is vital to carry out every body process. It carries almost all nutrients throughout your body, helps maintain temperature, flushes out all of the waste products, and lubricates between joints and organs. Most of our body weight consists of water, but don't deprive your body of water or else you may bloat. Be sure you eat enough fiber in your diet along with all the water you can drink (Kennedy . . . , 1987).

Eating Healthy

No fasting was involved during this program and it is suggested that you do not fast because your body needs good nutrition throughout the entire exercise program.

Here are some excellent foods for eating a good, healthy diet to re-fuel your muscles back to outstanding health again.

Breakfast	Lunch	Supper	Snacks
• Cereal	• Salad	• Steak	• Sunflower seeds
• Eggs	• Turkey	• Chicken	• Nuts
• Grits	• Chicken	• Seafood	• Popcorn
• Oatmeal	• Hamburger	• Pastas	• Fruit
• Toast	• Cheese	• Turkey	• Salads with olive oil
• Bacon	• Potatoes	• Hamburger	• Cheese and
• Grapefruit	• Cole slaw	• Lasagna	crackers
• Milk	• Broccoli	• Greens	• Occasional sweets
• Banana	• Greens	• Vegetables	• Protein drinks
• Waffles	• Beans	• Rice	• Protein bars
• Pancakes	• Bread	• Rolls	• Sandwiches
• Sausage	• Yogurt	• Bread	• Egg whites
• English muffins	• Fruit	• Desserts	• Chip and dip
• Buttermilk	• Vegetables	• Yogurt	• Etc.
• Orange juice	• Seafood	• Fruit	
• Syrup	• Etc.	• Jell-O	
• Etc.		• Etc.	

Eat plenty of carbs on your rest days and you'll really feel the difference in your strength when you resume exercises. These foods are excellent sources for all of the nutrients you'll need to eat the proper diet that will prosper you back into vigorous health again!

CHAPTER 13

Get Ready To Exercise

If you've ever heard the saying, "What do you think I'm doing this for, my health?" Well, this time you really are and the stakes are high. I Timothy 4:8 says, "For bodily exercise profiteth little: but godliness is profitable unto all things, having promise of the life that now is, and of that which is to come."

Bodily exercise can only profit in this life and not the life to come because we'll have spiritual bodies then. Even the Lord says that bodily exercise is profitable in this life. Those who have FMS, MPS, CFS, CFIDS, GWS or AA need all the profit in this life that they can get.

Exercise is profitable to us in several ways:

Table

- Gives more energy
- Helps relieve stress/cope with stress
- Helps to fight fatigue
- Helps against anxiety and depression
- Relaxes the body all over
- Improves ability to fall asleep
- Allows deeper sleep
- Tones muscles
- Improves heart rate
- Improves heart and lung condition
- And many more
  (Various sources)

- Burns calories
- Increases overall fitness
- Reduces risk of heart attacks/strokes
- Helps to control weight
- Increases flexibility
- Lowers blood pressure
- Raises HDL "good" cholesterol
- Improves circulation

I was always told that it's harder to regain your health than to maintain good health. I've also heard that prevention is the best cure. The Bible says in Proverbs 17:22 that "A merry heart doeth good like a medicine: but a broken spirit drieth the bones." A merry heart and exercise is like taking a natural anti-depressant. A merry heart and laughter stimulates the endorphins and helps to rid the body of disease.

Not only should we stay merry but we must also keep faith, hope, and charity alive. Stay happy and joyful, especially throughout this entire program. This program should cause you to be joyful and merry in your heart because of the mere fact that you're going to get some healing from virtually all of your symptoms of your condition(s). Not only that but rejoice in the fact that it is actually made available to you here and now. That alone should be enough to make you leap for joy.

I've also heard the saying that an ounce of prevention is worth a pound of cure. The Catch 22 about FMS and these other conditions is that not only do we not know how to prevent them, but we don't even know exactly what causes them. But have hope because I believe that many researchers and physicians will look into this program and find out more information than they've ever known about these conditions and also what happens to the muscles and connective tissues by further in-depth studies.

In order to understand how I found out this program really worked, I'll take you back to the time that I said that prayer several years ago. How God told me to "Only Just Believe." I kept thinking to myself that that's the hardest thing in the world to do . . . "Only Just Believe." To me, only just believing wasn't good enough. I guess I was expecting to be told to do some spectacular thing just like Naaman did, or that I would have to wait for a certain type of medication to be formulated for FMS etc . . . . By the way, I remember distinctively that I was also praying that I could stop taking all of those medications that I was on, too. Eventually the answer to that prayer came to pass after a few short years.

The following table shows the progress that I've made with this program versus all of the other programs that were prescribed to me.

- Prescribed program used drugs
- My program is natural: natural exercises, natural diet, and natural breathing with no cover-ups through medication(s).

SYMPTOMS	THEIR PROGRAM	THIS PROGRAM
Sleep Disorder	stayed the same or only improved with medication	improved but not yet 100%
Constant Muscle Pain	stayed the same	complete relief
Tension	relief for short time except when using medication	relieved dramatically
Muscle Spasm	relief for short time	relieved dramatically
Tender Points	tender points still present	gone for good

Trigger Points	trigger points still present	gone for good
Anxiety (panic) Attacks	no major change except with medication	improved dramatically
Headache	same except for narcotic pain relievers	improved but not yet 100%
Concentration	still poor	improved but not yet 100%
Memory	still poor	improved but not yet 100%
Energy Level	no change, still poor	improved but not yet 100%
Remission	No	Yes
Use medication	Yes	No

Figure 13-1: Comparison chart.

I noticed that the results of this evaluation seriously outweighed the treatment modalities that are said to be of standard treatment. Maybe one day this program will replace all of those others. A good rehabilitation or physical therapist could really appreciate this type of program. It does require some time but it is the most effective program that can deliver these dramatic results.

I also read in James 1:17 that, "Every good gift and every perfect gift is from above and cometh down from the Father of lights, with whom is no variableness, neither shadow of turning." So by this we can say that this program is a good and perfect gift and has come from above. After all, it started with a prayer and it will be finished with an answer to that prayer.

Since you are planning on using the weight lifting technique (anaerobic exercise), you will most definitely want to get a thorough checkup from your doctor before starting. You will also need a proper fitting weight lifting belt. You will have to go to a quality sporting goods store to buy a high quality weightlifting belt. Try them on until you find the right one for you. There are many quality weightlifting belts to choose from on the market today. Then, when you start, remember to take it easy. Safety is the most important thing.

Muscle growth is caused by microscopic tears in the muscle which in turn heal up to make more muscle mass.

And since muscles grow and repair during your sleep, remember to make sure you get extra sleep and rest. You're not as healthy as you used to be; like getting up at 6:30 a.m. every morning, eating breakfast, working for 8 hours, coming home, taking care of the kids, running three miles after playing basketball, going shopping, then reading and studying in the evening before bed time. That's too much if you have one of these illnesses.

Right now you're just not able to do all of that in one day if you truly have any of these conditions. I know from experience. Only after this program can I even come close to living that kind of life. Now that much is true.

Every day, at least 60 minutes before you start exercising take 100 mg of CO-Q-10. This will help give your body a boost and to use oxygen more efficiently. It allows your natural vitality to manifest itself. Even after this program, CO-Q-10 can really help keep your endurance and speed up. Many doctors advise FMS, MPS and CFS etc . . . patients to take it.

Also, take a one day supply of Ginkgo biloba at this time. You want to use the minimum dosage only. This will help dilate the blood vessels and I believe it will help allow nutrients and oxygen to get to the cells as well as help remove waste from the cells. It also helps counteract on any micro muscular disturbance.

It's going to be hard at first fighting the fatigue so make sure you get this right the first time around. Eight weeks will be a lot of valuable time wasted if you don't do everything just right the first time around. All you have to do is workout about 24 times and then reap all of the rewards of better health year after year for the rest of your life. And you can't really put a price on you and your health, because that's priceless. You may want to request that your physician give you leave from work so that you can follow through with this 8-week comprehensive program.

You know, I finally got really tired of feeling sick and tired. Through frustration and determination is how I found out that this program really works. During my three months of training I didn't know right off the bat that I was healed from most of the symptoms of these conditions. It came later when I got a check-up on my muscles. Some may call that serendipity. I just simply did not have constant pain, tender points or trigger points anymore, and neither were my muscles painful to the touch anymore. If this is what you want, then stick to the program.

Try to get rid of all your stressors and drop everything else that you're doing so you can focus on working your muscles every other day. Remember in about eight weeks you should be so much better and then you can take it easy and even stop the anaerobic exercise once your muscle problems are all gone and you do not feel anymore pain. Some will get relief in less than the recommended 8 weeks.

Since I no longer have trigger points, tender points, muscle stiffness, muscle tension nor constant muscle pain, the physicians agree that I no longer have the primary signs and/or symptoms of Fibromyalgia or these other conditions. Even though my sleep has not exactly gotten back to 100% normal, it has greatly improved to as high as 90%, along with my concentration, memory and energy levels. These symptoms may be residual from FMS, MPS, CFS or AA which were my primary diagnoses. Keep in mind that some believe FMS, MPS and CFS are all one and the same.

When a person is in pain, the pain sends transmitted signals back to the brain via nerves to produce endorphins (pain killers). These pain-killing endorphins are produced in order to block transmission and perception of pain. Some are as strong as opiate painkillers.

Weight training causes the body to release endorphins (naturally occurring morphine—like substances) which can lead to mood elevation.

Once all of your constant pain stops, your brain and nervous system might finally get a little rest from having to send those indefinite signals. Signals that you are in pain cause your brain to constantly react to send signals back to the origin site to help reduce that pain. This must really use a lot of electrical activity compared to a normal person who is not in constant pain.

Today medical research has been studying and showing that elderly people really get great benefits with weightlifting (strength training) too. And we're talking about 60, 70, 80 and 90 year olds. Surely the younger generation should be performing some type of strength training exercise as well. Most women were used to lifting weights at some time in their lives, mostly when they carried their babies around. Groceries and diaper bags add up to carrying weight around all day too.

Before jumping right into exercising I have tried to build you a foundation for you to stand on before I can just tell you what to do. You need to know why you're doing what you're doing. I'm sure you're beginning to understand. Like I'm telling you, in less than eight weeks hopefully you will be all finished and never need to do this program again. Fair enough?

Those patients suffering from FMS, MPS, CFS, GWS or AA could be helped immensely if not totally cured from these illnesses by simply following this comprehensive program that I've outlined in this book. But remember you must follow the program religiously every day until you are totally free from the pain and symptoms. When you compare how long you've been suffering from these illnesses, eight weeks really doesn't sound like a very long time at all, does it?

CHAPTER 14

The Proper Regimen

Amazingly enough, some people are still able to manage going to school or to work a job while they have FMS, MPS, CFS, GWS or AA. Others are completely debilitated and can't do either. But it may be better for you not to work a job or go to school while you are working through this program. The exercise regimen contained in this chapter may seem too vigorous at first glance and may leave you completely overwhelmed. But before you fall over in your chair you must remember that even before a baby can walk he must first learn to crawl. And so it is with this program. Be sure to bring your book with you to your workouts to follow the exercises correctly and in the proper chronological order. If you're not going to take the whole book with you at least take a copy of the workout list in appendix B and place it into a plastic sheet protector to protect it from moisture. It is highly recommended that you perform these exercises in the order they are in. Remember that you don't have to be in a rush and go through the program fast. Go slow and concentrate on the exercise at hand. And when you're done with one exercise turn the page and focus on the next one.

It is probably best not to start exercising first thing in the morning since muscle stiffness in most patients seems to be at its worst.

Where Can I Go To Exercise?

Health and fitness clubs, spas, schools, universities, YMCA, weight lifting gyms (bodybuilding gyms), community centers, home gyms, physical rehabilitation centers (usually must be prescribed by a physician), hotel/motel gym rooms and even your own home.

Aerobic Exercise

The first exercise you'll need to perform is aerobic exercise. Aerobic exercise is exercise that allows you to continually deliver oxygen to the muscles being used during the exercise. Aerobic exercises help strengthen your heart and lungs (cardiorespiratory system). In order for this to work, you must increase your pulse rate up to approximately 75% to 80% of your heart rate. Then you must continue this exercise for twenty minutes or more. Do not go over 45 minutes because this will tend to burn off muscle tissue. Aerobic exercises can also help burn off fat because it will increase the production of enzymes that change fat to energy. When we say aerobic exercise, people automatically think that they must bounce around like dancers, risking joint injuries, but that's not the only aerobic exercise there is. Stationary bicycles, rowing machines, stair climbing machines, treadmills, recumbent bicycles, electric steppers and cross country ski machines are also excellent examples of aerobic exercise equipment. An important note is that while performing aerobic exercise you should always be able to carry on a normal conversation. Many physicians prescribe aerobic exercise but the truth of the matter is that aerobic exercise alone doesn't seem to give any permanent relief from these illnesses. It only helps you get into better shape. And of course you'll need to do that in order to prepare for anaerobic exercises.

> *This program is almost like getting a flu shot. You feel a little sick for a short while after, but you don't get sick with the real sickness any at all (which could be ten times more devastating).*
>
> *R.D.G.*

When trying to figure out your target heart rate, use 220 heart beats per minute (BPM) as 100% of your maximum heart rate. Take the 220 and minus your age (let's say 35): 220 - 35 = 185 BPM. Multiply 185 BPM x 70% (.70) which will equal 129.5 BPM. You may divide this by 6 which will equal approximately 21.5 beats per 10 seconds on your watch. Most health and fitness spas have charts on their walls to help you find your target heart rate.

In this program you will need to develop your progress in stages. So let's find out starting with Stage I.

Stage I

Exercise with a stationary bicycle, treadmill or any other quality piece of aerobic exercise equipment for 5 to 10 minutes each day. You will need to rest on Saturday and Sunday. If you exercise Tuesday through Saturday, then rest on Sunday and Monday. If you are in fairly good shape it may take you just the first week to get in shape. Others may need to continue for another week or even more to get a little more fit. There's no rush; just be consistent.

When you find yourself recovering with ease from these exercises after a week or more, then you may move on to Stage II. Be extremely cautious from overdoing it too fast. That may only lead to more bedtime. And you don't want to keep stepping into that same old mud hole.

Stage II

While continuing Stage I exercises, exchange one day for a 15 to 20 minute aerobic workout instead of 5-10 minutes. When you feel you have recovered well, perform another 15 to 20 minute workout on another exercise day. Slowly work this increase up to the point that you are able to perform aerobic activity for 20 minutes per workout on a lot of your workout days. After sufficient progress, you may move on to Stage III.

Stage III

Anaerobic exercises

You are now ready to start anaerobic exercises. Anaerobic exercise does not allow you to continuously supply oxygen to the muscles during the exercise. You must stop to allow the muscles to recuperate. Weight lifting is a perfect example of anaerobic exercise. However, you will need to perform 15 minutes of aerobic exercise prior to anaerobic exercises in order to sufficiently warm up the muscles and to help prevent injury.

The benefits of anaerobic exercise are so astonishing that they're out of this world. Aside from those just listed, anaerobic exercise has been medically proven to:

- Increase muscular strength
- Tone and build muscle
- Increase metabolic rate (even at rest)
- Strengthen heart
- Decrease body fat percentage
- Decrease total serum cholesterol
- Increase HDL (good cholesterol)
- Lower blood pressure
- Increase neurochemical production (endorphins, etc.)
  (Various sources)

Anaerobic exercise has far outweighed aerobic exercise especially after relieving trigger points, tender points, constant widespread musculoskeletal pain, fatigue, insomnia and panic attacks.

These benefits have either been seriously overlooked by the fibromyalgic community or have just never been explored, studied and proven to this program's extent. Some studies were done on the effects of exercise in FMS, MPS, CFS, GWS and AA patients, but none proved that they could get as good of results as this program. Did you know that Rehabilitation centers often use weightlifting (anaerobic exercises) for rehabilitating injured patients? Sure. When people have nerve injuries or spinal injuries, what do the medical professionals typically recommend? Of course, it's weightlifting for rehabilitation, that's what. Those who lift weights seem to recover faster from injuries than those who do not. Without doubt, anaerobic exercise is the most beneficial of all exercises when speaking of and to the Fibromyalgic community. Anaerobic exercise obviously helps so much in health and injury that it should not be shunned without serious consideration by those who have such problems, until they have given their best effort to try it. In other words, don't knock it till you try it. If you have other disabilities that limit how much exercise you can do, then just target those areas that you want relieved. Even if it's just for the arms, neck and shoulder areas. Refer to the areas of relief for each exercise to determine which ones you'll need to perform.

Reps stands for repetitions. Each time you perform a weight lifting exercise, from the starting position to the end position and then back to the starting position, is one *rep*. When you perform 12-15 *reps*, one immediately after the other and then stop for a rest that is called a *set*.

Please note that you are to wait exactly 60 seconds between each set with this program. The 60 second wait is vitally important for oxygen recuperation to your muscles, so get a quality watch that counts the seconds clearly.

Finding your weight. You will find your perfect weight level for each exercise by picking a certain weight to test and see how many *reps* you can perform. If you don't get up to 12 *reps*, go to a lighter weight. On the other hand, if you can perform more than 15 *reps*, you need to use a heavier weight. Your correct weight will allow you to perform between 12 and 15 *reps*.

After you find your weight, it's a relief to know that the weight you've just found is strictly for you and not anybody else. The bottom line is that you can do these exercises reasonably well because they are based solely on your muscle strength and not someone else's. This is where the fear of weight lifting exercise diminishes. Plus you are going to start out with a lower weight than your own weight level; you will not need to go to your maximum weight level until the final stages and by then you will be so much stronger that it shouldn't even seem hard.

The Warm Up Exercise will help to sufficiently heat up muscles to prepare you for anaerobic exercises and to help prevent any injuries.

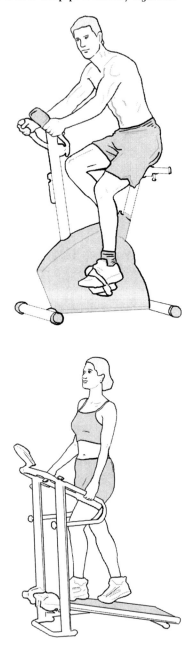

Figure 14-1: Aerobic Exercise.
Perform at least 10-15 minutes before starting anaerobic exercises.

Starting the Anaerobic Routine

After warming up with aerobic exercises for about 15 minutes, move on to the weight lifting routine. It is very important that you do not allow your body to cool down too much before you start your anaerobic exercise since this helps to prevent injuries. 1 to 5 minutes will be plenty of rest time before lifting weights.

Always use a quality weightlifting belt before lifting any weights. However some exercises may not permit you to comfortably wear a belt, like the crunch and sometimes the hyperextension, etc. The following exercises are designed to eliminate tender points and trigger points throughout the whole body. See Figure 2-3 and 2-4 for tender point locations. See Figures 3-1 through 3-11 for most trigger point locations. Weightlifting helps to tighten tendons which in turn will help reduce hypermobility in joints, a condition that is not uncommon with these syndromes. Weightlifting also helps reduce pain levels by increasing endorphins which also help Stage IV sleep. Then you'll be able to get to sleep easier and have deeper sleep for better recuperation and new muscle growth.

Stage IV

In Stage IV you are performing weight lifting exercise. In order to start out easy, pick a lower weight than what your weight level is and perform 1 set of 7 *reps* for each exercise. Always rest from anaerobic exercises for at least one full day before working out again. Example: lift weights on Monday, rest Tuesday, and then weight lift again on Wednesday and Friday, and so on.

Still keep the aerobic activity up on days you don't lift. An important note is that the aerobic exercise for warming up and cooling down on days you perform anaerobic exercise is sufficient enough to count as aerobic exercise for that day. So to get this exactly right, you will be performing aerobic exercise 5 days a week but performing anaerobic exercises only 3 days of those five days with 2 days rest in between each week. (See calendar).

	Sunday	Monday	Tuesday	Wednesday	Thursday	Friday	Saturday
Aerobic exercise		Warm-up ✓ and Cool Down	✓	Warm up ✓ and Cool Down	✓	Warm up ✓ and Cool Down	
Anaerobic exercise		✓		✓		✓	
Rest	✓						✓

Stage V

After you are able to recover from 1 set of 7 *reps* of each exercise, increase to 2 sets of 7 reps for each exercise; Still keeping the aerobic activity in tack. After good progress is made move on to Stage VI.

Stage VI

You are now ready to weight lift performing 1 set of 15 *reps* for each exercise at your highest weight level. And you must still keep the aerobic exercise going. After sufficient progress is made, move on to Stage VII.

Stage VII

You are now ready for the final stage. Perform 2 sets of 15 *reps* for each exercise at your highest found weight level while keeping the aerobic exercise in tack with some advanced sprinting (to be discussed), and continue for up to 8 weeks. After completing this stage all tender points, trigger points, and virtually all constant widespread musculoskeletal pain will have vanished. My wish is that you prosper to be in better health from this program. You are welcome to discontinue the anaerobic exercise after completing Stage VII now.

See the muscles of the body that will receive great benefits of relief.

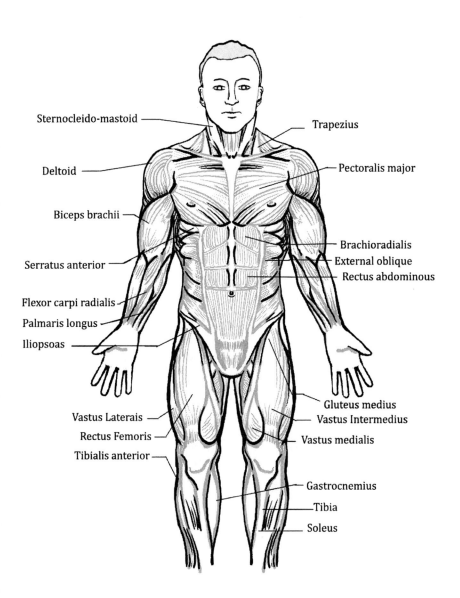

Figure 14-2A: Muscles of the Body; Front view.

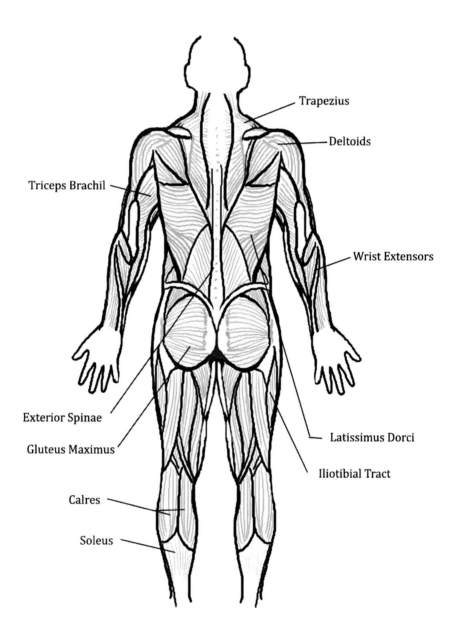

Figure 14-2B: Muscles of the Body; Backview.

The following are all of the exercises you must perform. Perform all of them according to the stage level you are in.

Exercise #1

The Squat

The squat really works the quadriceps (thighs), the hamstrings and the gluteus muscles. Using your weight level get your heels on a safe board (about 1" to 2" above the ground) and bring the weights up above your shoulders. Slowly squat down to a comfortable position and then come back up to the standing position. Do not try to squat down too low. Some do not like to use anything under the heels. By performing flat-footed this will help the gluteus muscles even more.

Note: By using dumbbells you will avoid possible back injury because you will not have the bar across your back. Be sure to use something safe and sturdy under your heels (optional) and wear your weightlifting belt. Using dumbbells, find your weight level and perform.

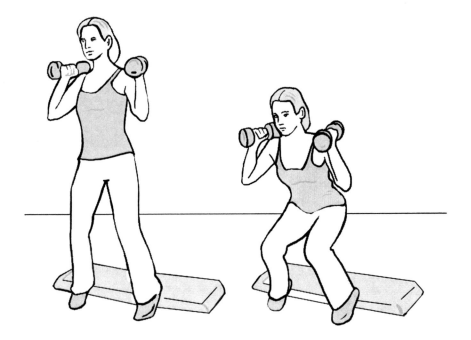

Figure 14-3A: The Squat.
Areas of relief: quadriceps, femoris, gluteus muscles,
hamstrings, all knee and hip extensors.

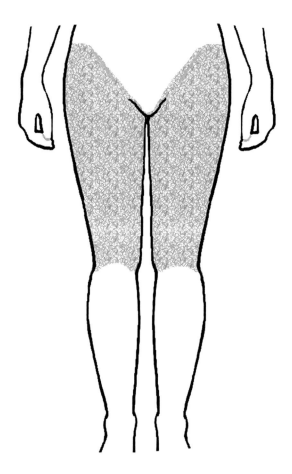

Figure 14-3B: Areas of trigger point and tender point relief from the squat.

Exercise #2A

The Leg Curl

The leg curl really helps the hamstrings. Using a machine, set it to your weight level using a pin in the weight blocks and lie face down on the bench. Putting the back of your heels against the pads and holding the handles with your hands, bring the back of your heels closer to your bottom (about as far as the travel will let you) and then let down again slowly.

Using a machine, find your weight and perform according to your stage level.

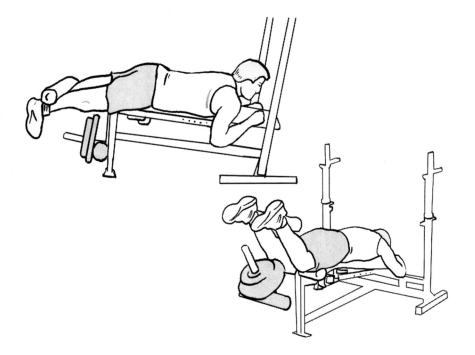

Figure 14-4A: The Leg Curl.

Areas of relief: hamstrings

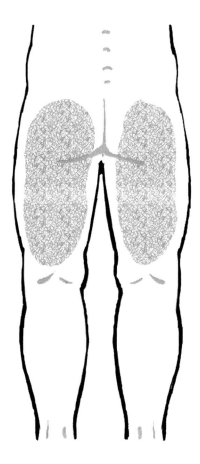

Figure 14-4B: Areas of trigger point and tender point relief from the Leg Curl.

Exercise #2B

The Leg Curl Variation

One of the latest leg curl variations can be used in place of the previous exercise. There are new machines out which have a leg curl variation and it's basically achieving the same thing. In fact, it may even be safer, since the thighs are in a 90° angle to the rest of the torso during the entire Leg Curl. It's a seated leg curl. This seems to help prevent back injuries better than other variations. Using a machine, find your weight and perform according to your stage level.

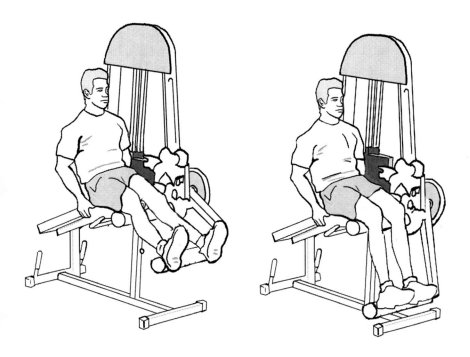

Figure 14-5A: The leg curl variation.

Areas of relief: hamstrings

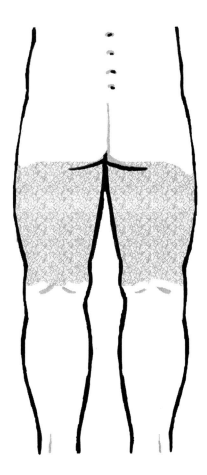

Figure 14-5B: Areas of trigger point and tender point relief from the Leg Curl variation.

Exercise #3

The Bench Press

The Bench Press is an excellent exercise to help build and strengthen your chest (pectoral) muscles. Find your weight with dumbbells and lie down on your back in the beginning position. Lower the weights down near your chest and then back up again.

Using dumbbells or a machine, find your weight and perform according to your stage level.

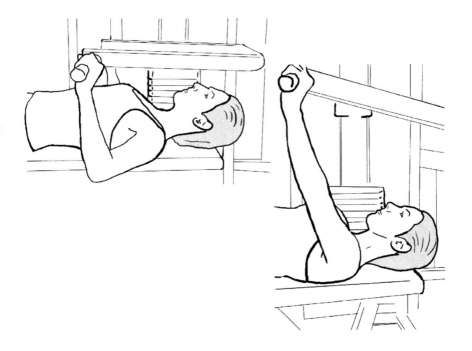

Figure 14-6A: The Bench Press.

Areas of relief: pectorals, deltoids, triceps

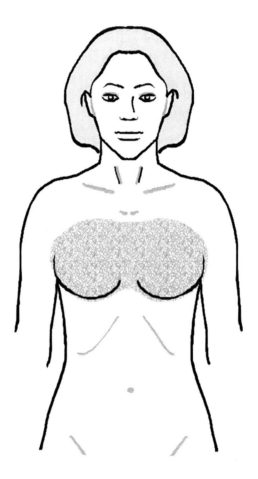

Figure 14-6B: Areas of trigger point and tender point relief from the Bench Press.

Exercise #4

The Overhead Barbell Press

The overhead Barbell Press helps to strengthen your deltoid muscles. Find your weight with dumbbells and sit on a bench in the beginning position. Raise the weights up as high as you can and lower back down to the beginning position. Find your weight and perform.

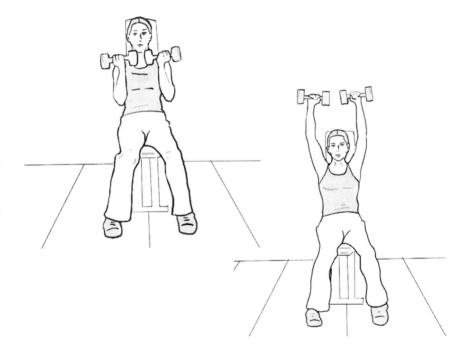

Figure 14-7A: The Overhead Barbell Press.

Areas of relief: Deltoids and triceps.

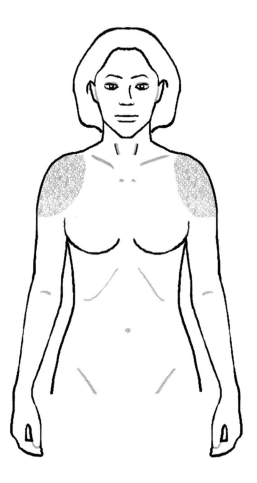

Figure 14-7B: Areas of trigger point and tender point relief from the Overhead Barbell Press.

Exercise #5

The Upright Row

The Upright Row helps strengthen muscles on top of the shoulders. Find your weight and let the dumbbells hang in front of you with your palms facing your thighs. Slowly lift them up all the way under your chin as though you were rowing a boat that way. See illustration.

Using dumbbells or a barbell, find your weight and perform according to your stage level.

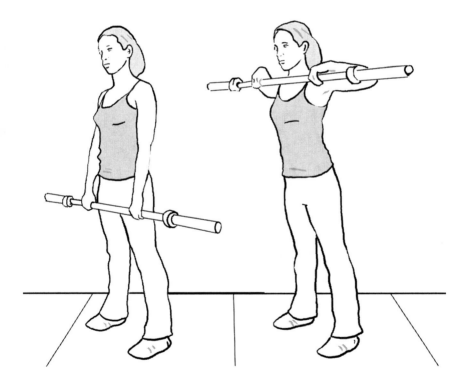

Figure 14-8A: The Upright Row.

Areas of relief: Deltoids, upper trapezius, stenocleido-mastoid, biceps, radialis.

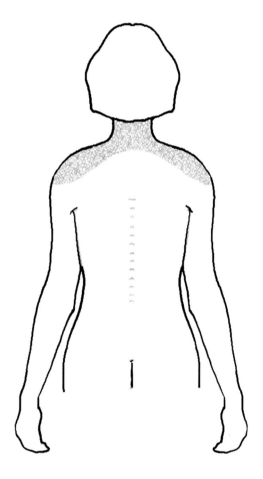

Figure 14-8B: Areas of trigger point and tender point relief from the Upright Row.

Exercise #6

Shrugs

Shrugs are easy. Find your weight and let your arms hang down with your palms facing your thighs. Simply shrug your shoulders upward and then back to beginning position.

Using dumbbells or barbells, find your weight and perform according to your stage level.

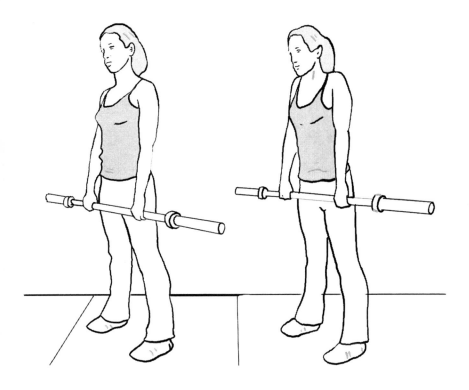

Figure 14-9A: The Shrug.

Areas of relief: Upper trapezius, deltoids, radialis, biceps, sternocleido-mastoid.

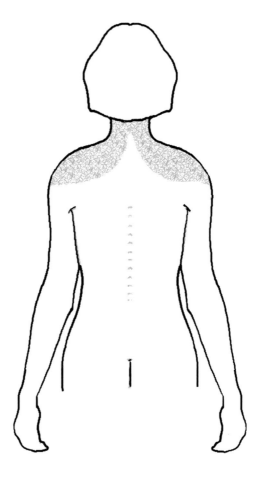

Figure 14-9B: Areas of trigger point and tender point relief from the Shrug.

Exercise #7

The Barbell Row

The Barbell Row really helps the upper and mid-back muscles. Find your weight and bend over forward, keeping your back level with the floor. Slowly pull weights up into the mid-stomach area and let back down again. It should almost feel like rowing a boat. Keep knees slightly bent.

Using a barbell or dumbbells, find your weight and perform according to your stage level.

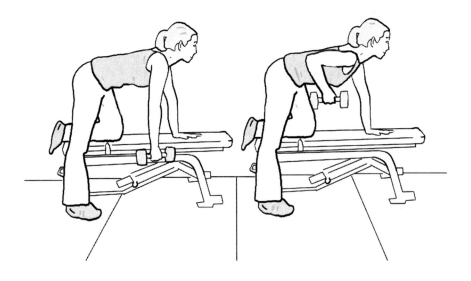

Figure 14-10A: The Barbell Row.

Areas of relief: Trapezius, rhomboids, and biceps.

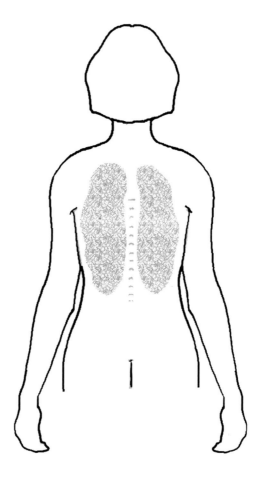

Figure 14-10B: Areas of trigger point and tender point relief from the Barbell Row.

Exercise #8

The Lat Pull Down

The Lat Pull Down works muscles in the upper back. Find your weight on a machine and hold the bar while getting into a sitting position. Pull the bar down in front of you until it comes near to your chest and then back up again.

Using a Lat bar on a machine perform according to your stage level.

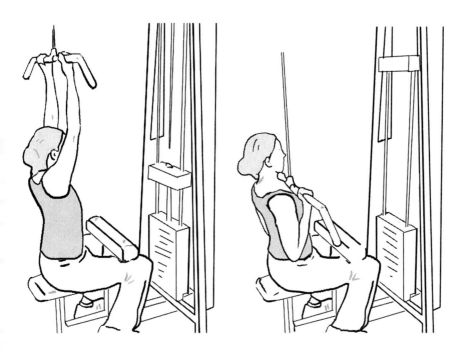

Figure 14-11A: The Lat Pull Down.

Areas of relief: Latissimus dorsi, rhomboids, and biceps.

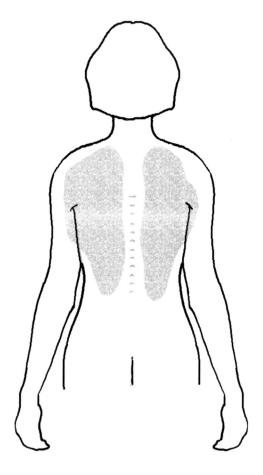

Figure 14-11B: Areas of trigger point and tender point relief from the Lat Pull Down.

Exercise #9

The Hyperextension or Low Back Machine

The Hyperextension or Low Back machine really helps to strengthen the lower back.

The Hyperextension can be performed on a Roman chair (not shown). Put your hands on the handrails and position yourself on the chair part and place the back of your heels under the leg pads. Let your body bend forward, placing your face closer to the floor. Then raise your upper body back up until your back is level with the floor, then go back down again.

The Back Machine variation can be used instead of the Roman chair. Set weight on machine and get into position. Lean back on the padded section as far as comfortable and then come forward again.

Using a Roman chair or machine, perform according to your stage level. The Roman chair does not require weights but uses your own body weight.

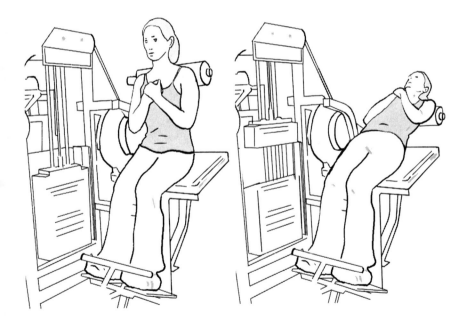

Figure 14-12A: The Hyperextension.

Areas of relief: Lower back.

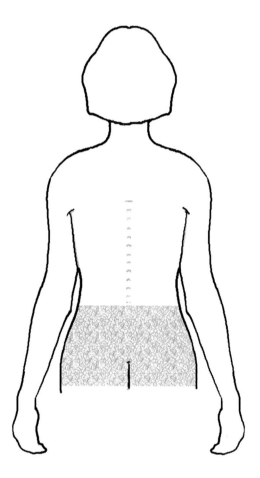

Figure 14-12B: Areas of trigger point and tender point relief from the Hyperextension.

Exercise #10

The Triceps Extension

The Triceps Extension helps the backs of the upper arms. Simply use a dumbbell, reaching up high and lowering the weight behind your head (being careful not to touch your head) and then back up again. You may want to support your arm just near the elbow with your other hand.

Using a dumbbell, find your weight for one arm at a time and perform your stage level.

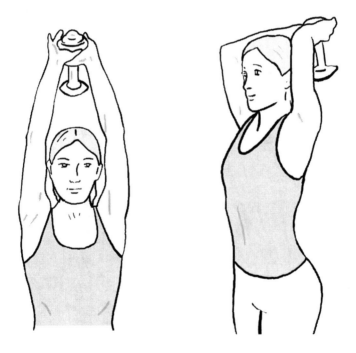

Figure 14-13A: The Tricep Extension.

Areas of relief: Triceps.

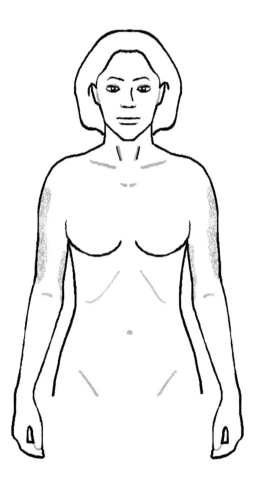

Figure 14-13B: Areas of trigger point relief from the Tricep Extension.

Exercise #11

The Barbell Curl

The Barbell Curl helps strengthen the front of the arms (biceps). Using a barbell or dumbbells, hold the weights downward with your palm facing outward in the beginning position. Curl the weights up toward your shoulders without moving your elbows from their original position and back down again.

Using a barbell or dumbbells, find your weight and perform your stage level.

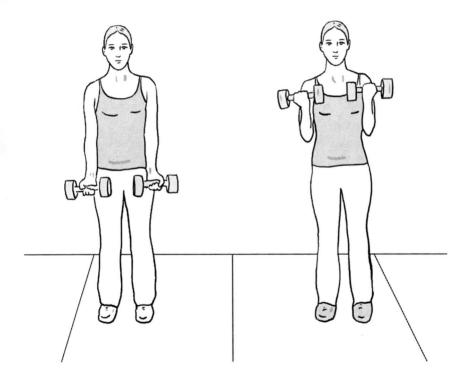

Figure 14-14A: The Barbell/Dumbbell Curl.

Areas of relief: Biceps.

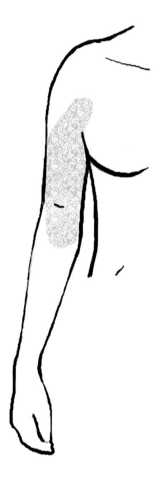

Figure 14-14B: Areas of trigger point and tender point relief from the Barbell Curl.

Exercise #12

The Reverse Curl

The Reverse Curl is similar to the regular curl but has the palms facing your thighs instead. Start in the beginning position and curl the weights up toward your shoulders and then back down again. This exercise will help to relieve a lot of tension in the forearms.

Using dumbbells or a barbell, find your weight and perform according to your stage level.

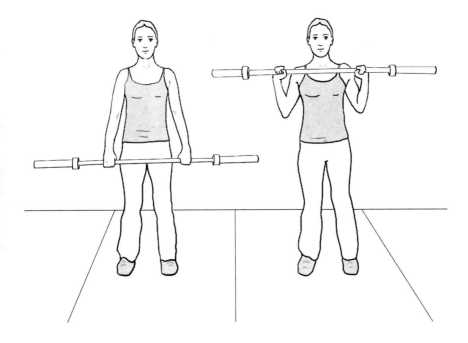

Figure 14-15A: The Reverse Curl.

Areas of relief: Biceps, radialis, brachioradialis, and wrist flexors.

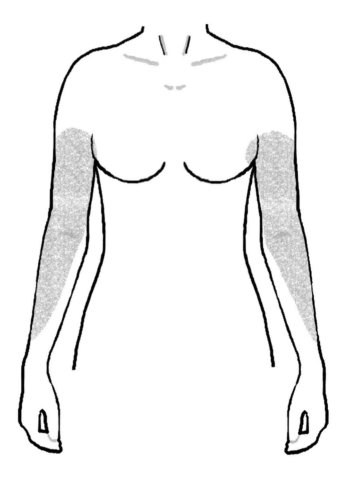

Figure 14-15B: Areas of trigger point and tender point relief from the Reverse Curl.

Exercise #13

The Wrist Curl and the Reverse Wrist Curl

The Wrist Curl curls the weights up with the palms facing up and the Reverse Wrist Curl curls the weights up with the palms facing down. These exercises help to relax the tension in the forearms also. While sitting, rest your arms on the top of your thighs for addtional support. Perform according to your stage level.

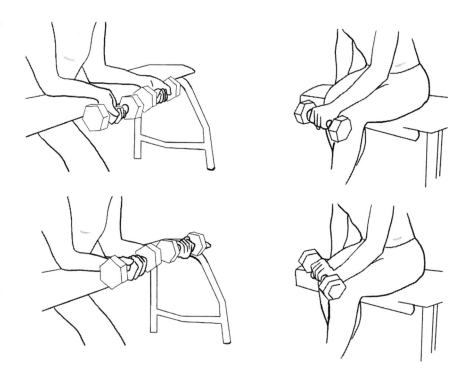

Figure 14-16A: The Wrist Curl and Reverse Wrist Curl.

Areas of relief: Wrist flexors of the forearm, extensors of the forearm.

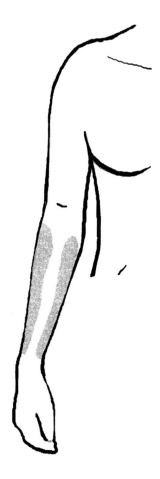

Figure 14-16B: Areas of trigger point and tender point relief from the Wrist Curl and the Reverse Wrist Curl.

Exercise #14

The Hand Grip Exercise

The Hand Grip Exercise helps to strengthen weak hands and also helps relieve tension in the hands. Use them in both hands at the same time for best results. Perform the Hand Grip Exercise according to your stage level.

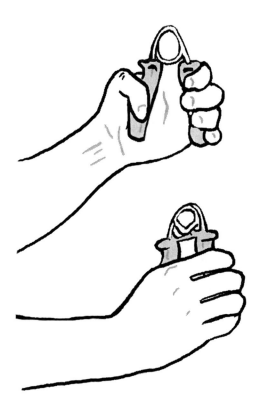

Figure 14-17A: The Hand Grip Exercise.

Areas of relief: Finger flexors.

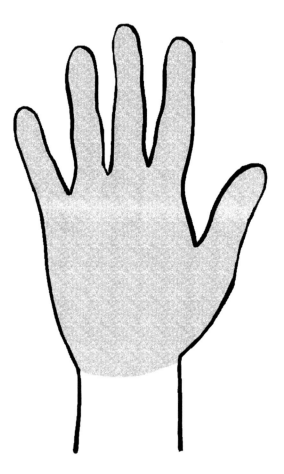

Figure 14-17B: Areas of trigger point relief from the Hand Grip Exercise.

Exercise #15

The Calf Raises or Toe Press

The Calf Raise or Toe Press really works the calves to make them strong. For the Calf Raise, use an elevated lift for the balls of your feet. Raise your body up to the point of standing on your tipped toes and back down again.

For the Toe Press use a leg press machine that you can press with the balls of your feet on the footing.

Using a machine, find your weight and perform according to your stage level.

Note: If you don't use a machine, perform them while standing up with no weights (on a lift).

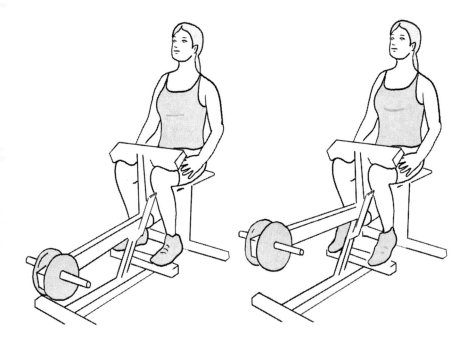

Figure 14-18A: The Calf Raise or Toe Press.

Areas of relief: Gastrocnemius and soleus.

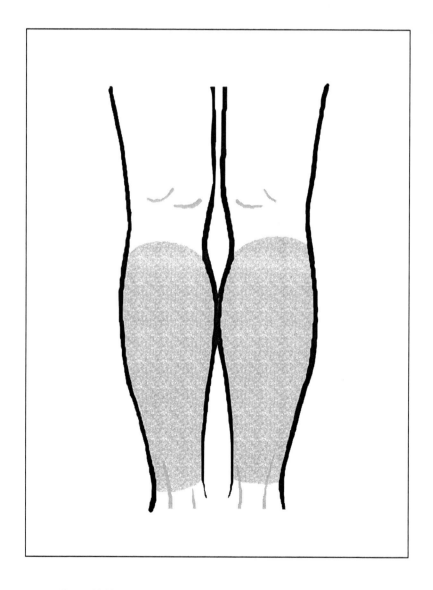

Figure 14-18B: Areas of trigger point relief from the Calf Raise or Toe Press.

Exercise #16

The Shin Exercise

The Shin Exercise really works because you can feel the burn in your shins after a good work out. Stand on your heels or an elevated support. With your toes hanging off of the support, raise them up so that you are standing on the heels of your feet and then down again.

Perform according to your stage level.

Note: Hold on to wall or support with your hands for additional support.

Begin:

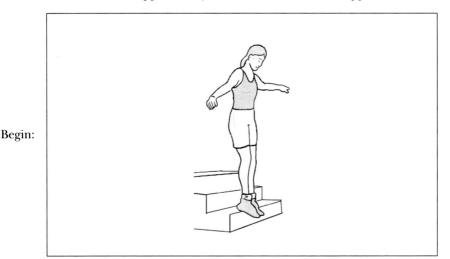

End:

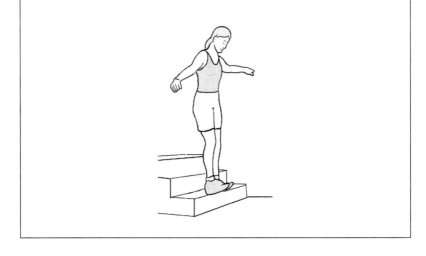

Figure 14-19A: The Shin Exercise.

Areas of relief: Shins.

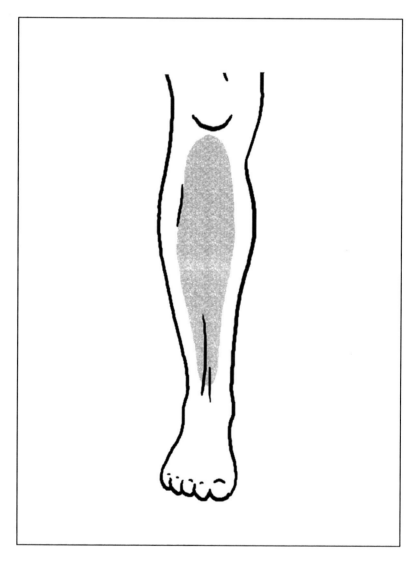

Figure 14-19B: Areas of trigger point relief from the Shin Exercise.

Exercise #17

The Toe Crunch and Toe Spread

The Toe Crunch and Toe Spread will help to relieve tension in the feet. Scrunch your toes as tight as a fist and then spread them out as far as you can. Perform according to your stage level.

Begin:

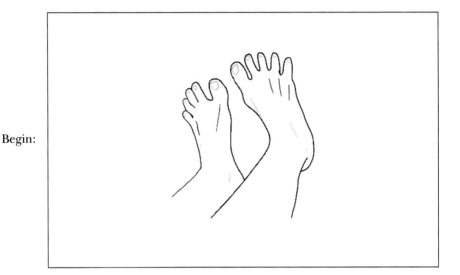

End:

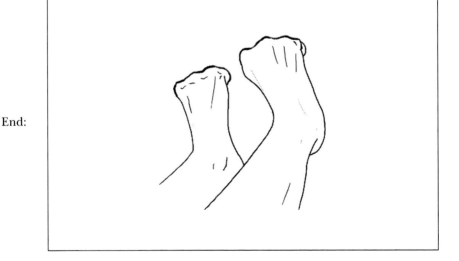

Figure 14-20A: The Toe Crunch and Toe Spread Exercises.

Areas of relief: Intrinsic foot muscles.

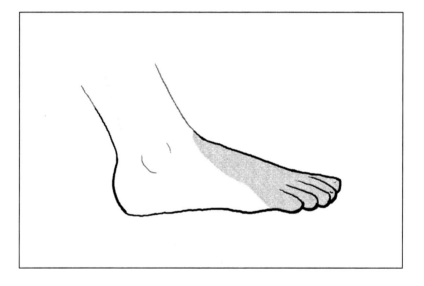

Figure 14-20B: Areas of trigger point relief from the Toe Crunch and Toe Spread Exercises.

Exercise #18

The Machine Crunch or Cross Crunch

The latest crunch machines can really help with the abdominal muscles.

Crunch machines have replaced the old sit up exercise. In order to use set the pin to your weight level and perform according to your stage level. If you can't find a crunch machine then lie down on a mat and bend your knees up to prepare for cross crunches. Place your left foot on top of your right knee (crossing your leg) and your finger tips on your temples. Slowly bring your right elbow up to your left knee touching it. After one set reverse your legs for the other side. Cross crunches are easier this way and much safer (including not placing your hands behind your head or neck). Using a machine find your weight and perform according to your stage level.

Note: If you can't use a crunch machine perform cross crunches.

Begin:

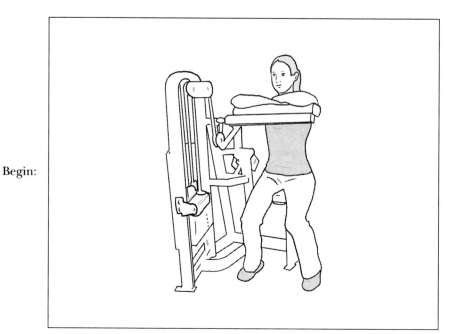

End:

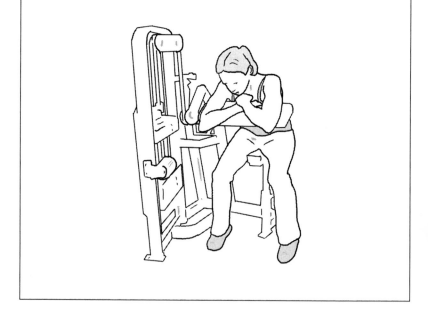

Figure 14-21A: The Machine Crunch/Cross Crunch.

Areas of relief: Abdominals, hip flexors, quadriceps, and obliques.

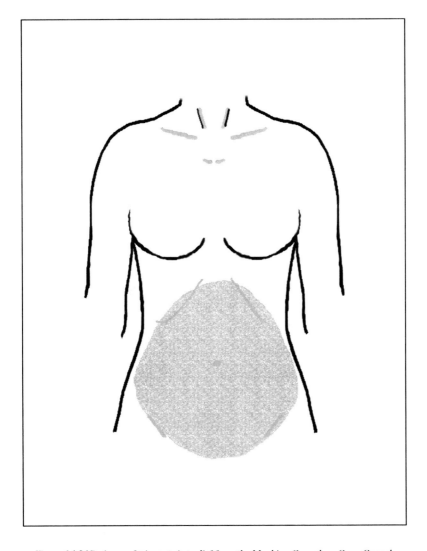

Figure 14-21B: Areas of trigger point relief from the Machine Crunch or Cross Crunch.

Exercise #19

The Alternate Leg Kick

The Alternate Leg Kick helps strengthen the lower abdominal muscles. Lean against a desk or table to where you almost sit on the edge and smoothly raise one leg up at a time and back down again, alternating from one leg to the other.

Using no weights, perform according to your stage level, alternating each leg kick. For best results, you should actually sit on the edge of your seat or desk.

Ankle weights can be used to help strengthen the lower abdominal muscles even better.

Begin:

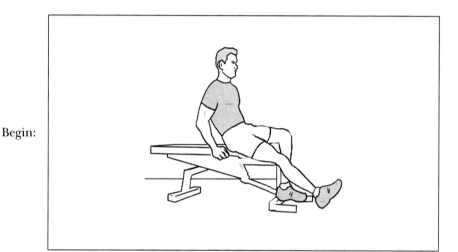

End:

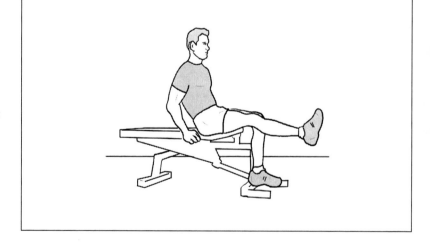

Figure 14-22A: The Alternate Leg Kick.

Areas of relief: Lower abdominals.

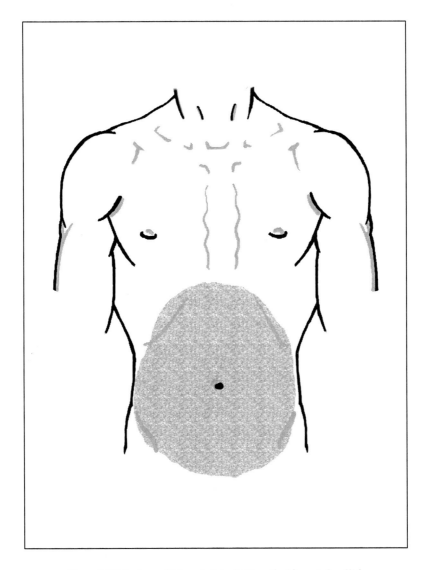

Figure 14-22B: Areas of trigger point relief from the Alternate Leg Kick.

Exercise #20

The Side Bends

Side Bends help strengthen the sides of your waist area. Using your weight level in one hand lower the weight downward and then straighten back to a straight position. Using a dumbbell, find your weight and perform according to your stage level. Perform on one side then alternate to the other side.

Begin:

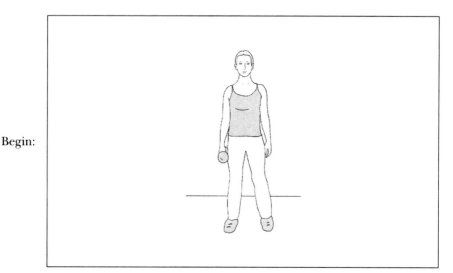

End:

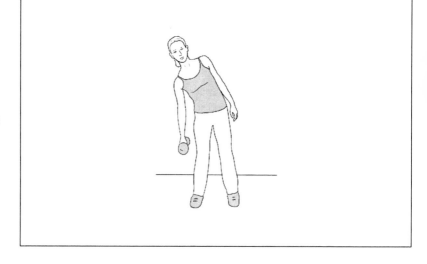

Figure 14-23A: The Side Bends.

Areas of Relief: Lateral flexors, erector spinae, and abdominals.

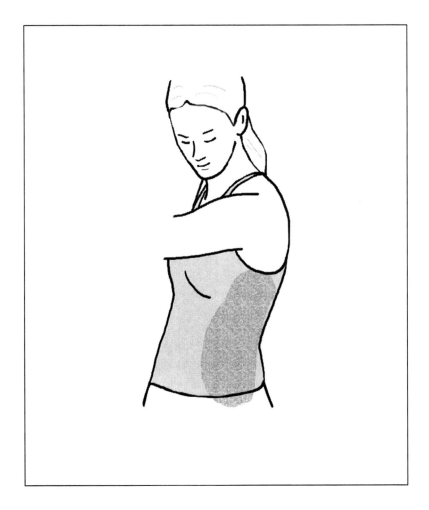

Figure 14-23B: Areas of trigger point relief from the Side Bends.

Exercise #21

The Right Side of the Neck Exercise

Important Note: The instructions for the following four (4) neck exercises should be read completely before actually starting the exercises. These neck exercises were used in the original program but they are considered optional. If you've been injured in your neck or for any reason you think you shouldn't do these exercises, ask your physician first. However, if you neglect these, you may not be able to get tender point, trigger point and pain relief.

The neck exercises will help with the neck pain, tender points and trigger points. Starting with the Right Side of the Neck, lie down on the left side of your body, keeping head clear off of the bench when you perform repetitions. Lower your head downward and then lift it back upward without turning your head to the left or right. Keep your eyes on a fixed object in front of you. Using no weights, perform according to your stage level.

Begin: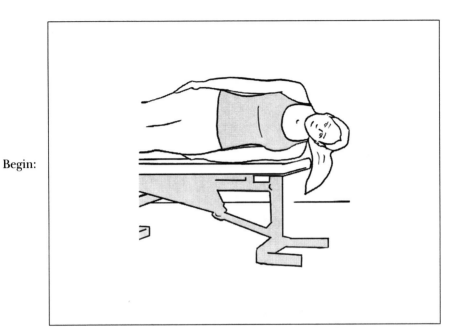

End: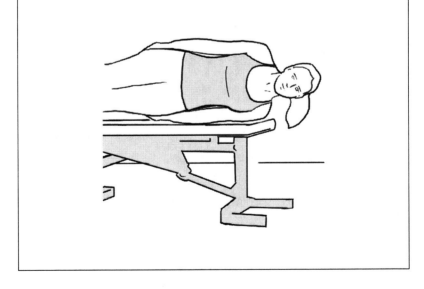

Figure 14-24A: The Right Side of the Neck Exercise.

Areas of Relief: The following four neck exercises for the neck give relief to the erector spinae, sterncleido-mastoid and superior fibers of the trapezium.

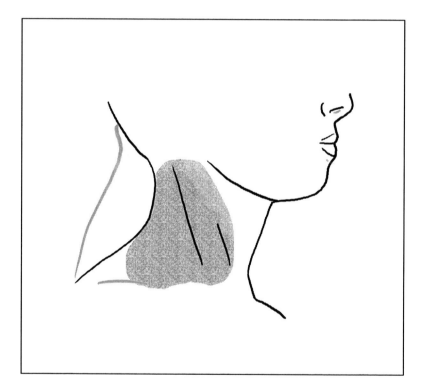

Figure 14-24B: Areas of trigger point and tender point relief from the Right Side of the Neck Exercises.

Exercise #22

The Left Side of the Neck Exercise

The left side of the neck should be done opposite of the right side. NOTE: Perform the Left side immediately after the Right and then start the count for 60 seconds. That's 1 *rep* for both sides. Using no weights, perform according to your stage level.

Begin:

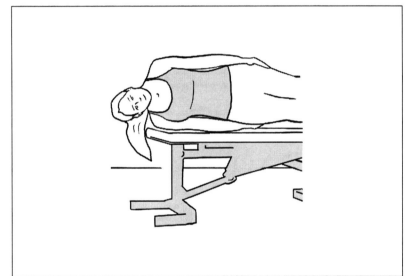

End:

Figure 14-25A: The Left Side of the Neck Exercise.

Areas of relief: Erector spinae, sternocleido-mastoid and superior fibers of the trapezium.

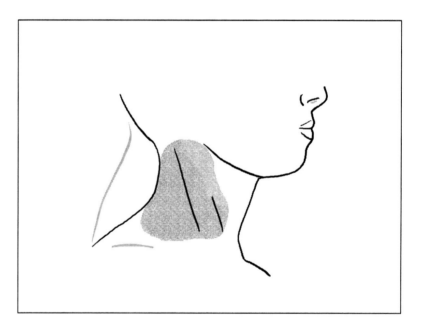

Figure 14-25B: Areas of trigger point and tender point relief from the left side of the Neck Exercise.

Exercise #23

The Front of the Neck

Important: Only perform the Front and Back of Neck exercises after the Right and Left Side of the Neck Exercises (e.g., right and left side of the neck, rest for 60 seconds, then front and back of the neck, rest for 60 seconds. Then right and left side again, then rest for 60 seconds and finally Front and Back of the Neck exercises and rest again.) That's two full sets. This will help keep the cervical vertebrae in a more proper alignment after exercising. Using no weights, perform according to your stage level.

Begin:

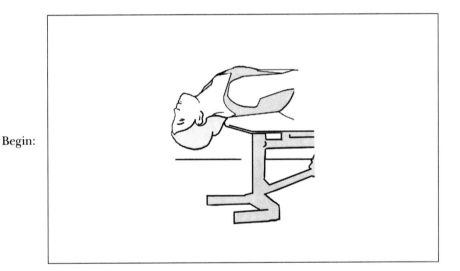

End:

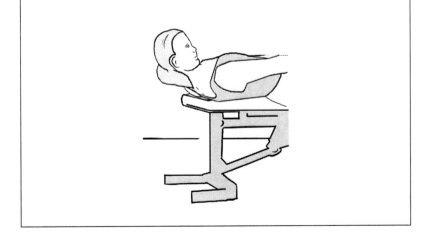

Figure 14-26A: The Front of the Neck Exercise.

Areas of relief: Erector spinae, sternocleido-mastoid, superior fibers of the trapezius.

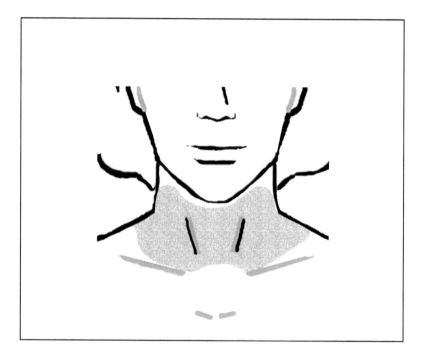

Figure 14-26B: Areas of trigger point and tender point relief from the Front of the Neck Exercise.

Exercise #24

The Back of the Neck Exercise

Note: Reread the instructions for Front and Back of the Neck Exercise under Front of the Neck Exercise. Using no weights, perform according to your stage level. Place hands under thighs for support.

Begin:

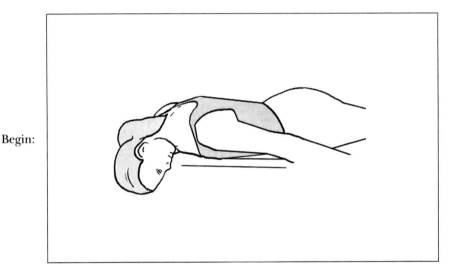

End:

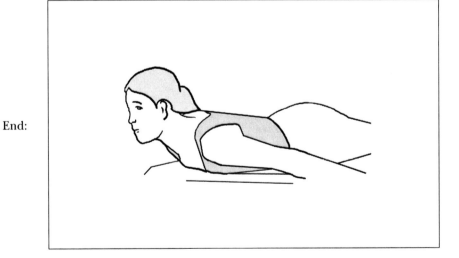

Figure 14-27A: The Back of the Neck Exercise.

Areas of relief: Erector spinae, sternocleido-mastoid, superior fibers of the trapezius.

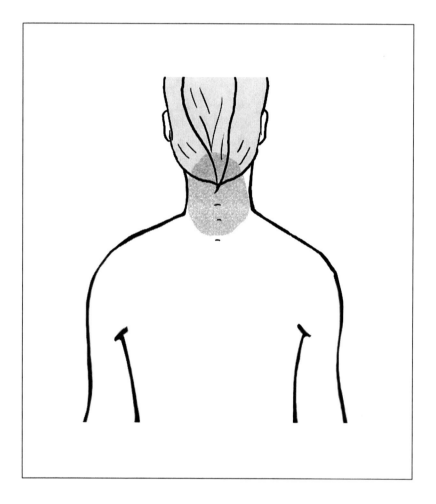

Figure 14-27B: Areas of trigger point and tender point relief from the Back of the Neck Exercise.

Exercise #25

The Eye Muscle Exercise

The eye exercises help remove trigger points from any of the extrinsic eye muscles. Simply cup your hands over your eyes and hold your hands steady, also supporting your face. Move only your eyes, looking up and down and then left to right. Perform reps and sets according to your stage level.

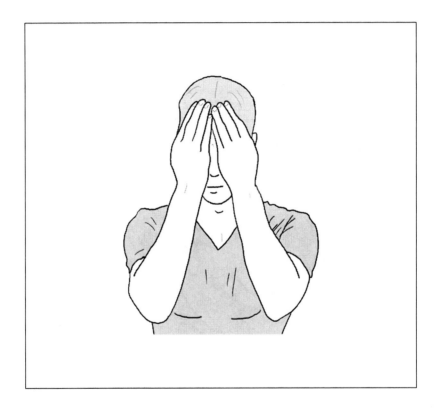

Figure 14-28A: The Eye Muscles Exercise.

Areas of relief: Extrinsic eye muscles.

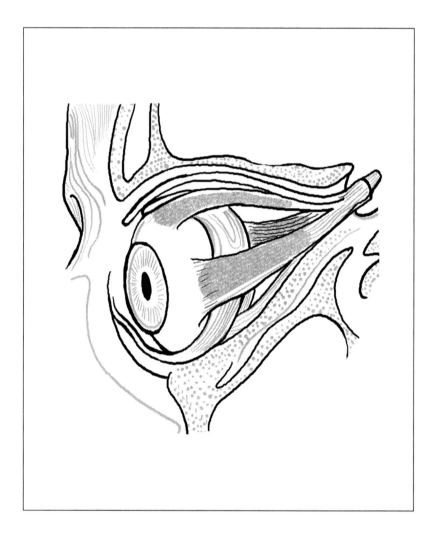

Figure 14-28B: Areas of trigger point relief from the Eye Muscle Exercise.

Exercise #26

The Pucker Exercise

The Pucker exercises help with tension in the facial muscles. Simply squinch your eyes shut as tightly as you can, as well as your forehead, nose and lips. Hold for 1 second and then open your mouth in a wide open expression including your eyes and forehead. Perform according to your stage level.

Begin:

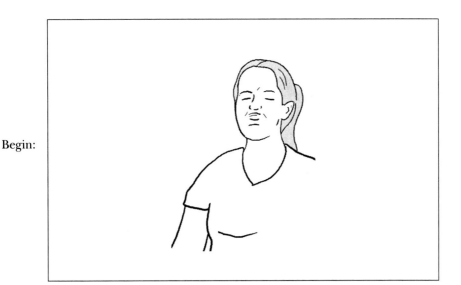

End:

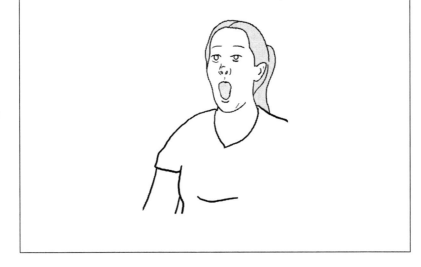

Figure 14-29A: The Pucker Exercise.

Areas of relief: Facial muscles.

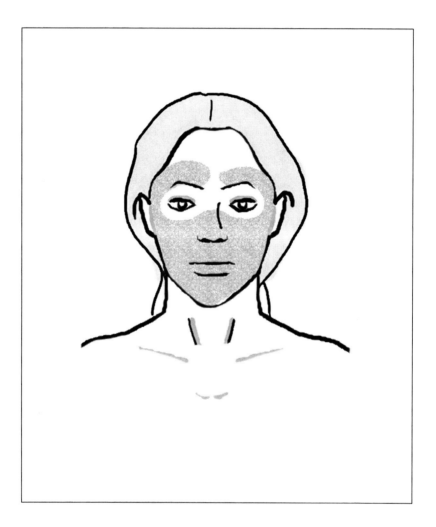

Figure 14-29B: Areas of trigger point relief from the Pucker Exercise.

Exercise #27

The Opening Jaw Exercise

The following two (2) jaw exercises will also help with TMJ. The Opening Jaw exercise will help with tension in the jaw muscles (including trigger points). Hold both thumbs under the front of your jaw and open holding resistance with your thumbs, then close again. Perform according to your stage level.

Begin:

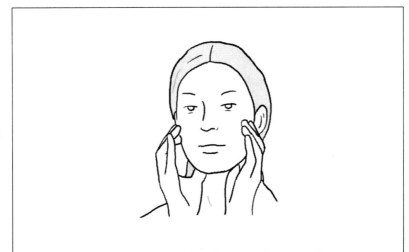

End:

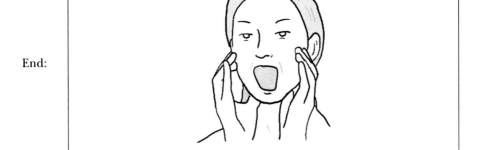

Figure 14-30A: The Opening Jaw Exercise.

Areas of relief: Jaw area.

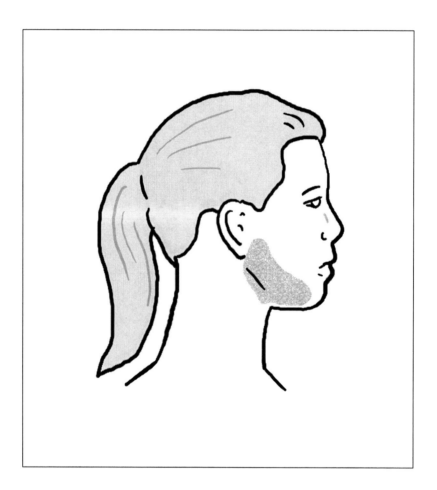

Figure 14-30B: Areas of trigger point relief from the Opening Jaw Exercise.

Exercise #28

The Closing Jaw Exercise

The Closing Jaw exercise is easy to perform. Wash hands first then open jaw slightly and put the 1st and 2nd fingers of both hands on top of your bottom row of teeth. Apply pressure as you open and then close your jaw. You'll find that your jaw muscles are very strong. Perform according to your stage level.

Begin:

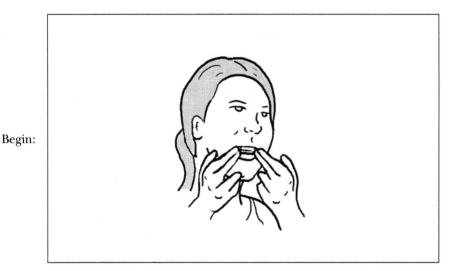

End:

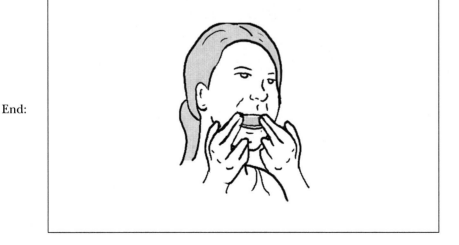

Figure 14-31A: The Closing Jaw Exercise.

Areas of relief: Jaw area.

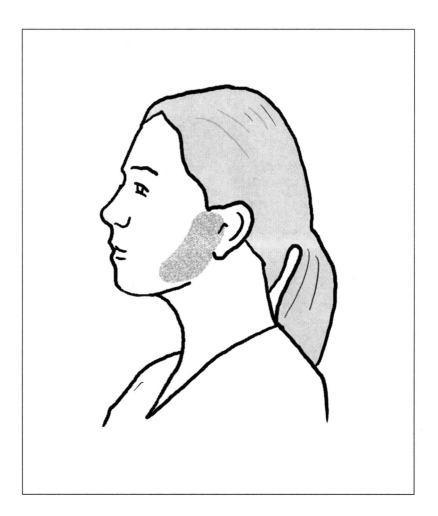

Figure 14-31B: Areas of trigger point relief from the Closing Jaw Exercise.

Exercise #29

The Fish Hook Exercise

The Fish Hook exercise helps with trigger points around the mouth and cheeks. Simply curl up your index fingers like a fish hook and hook them inside of your mouth and cheeks. Pull outward with your fingers and with some resistance use your mouth to pull your fingers back to the starting position. Perform according to your stage level.

Begin:

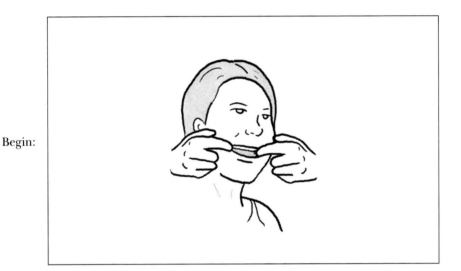

End:

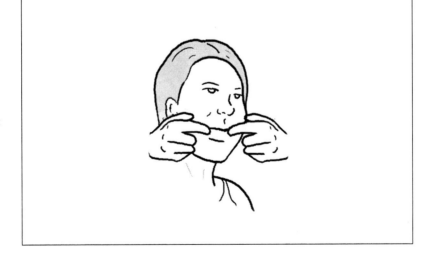

Figure 14-32A: The Fish Hook Exercise.

Areas of Relief: Mouth and Cheek muscles.

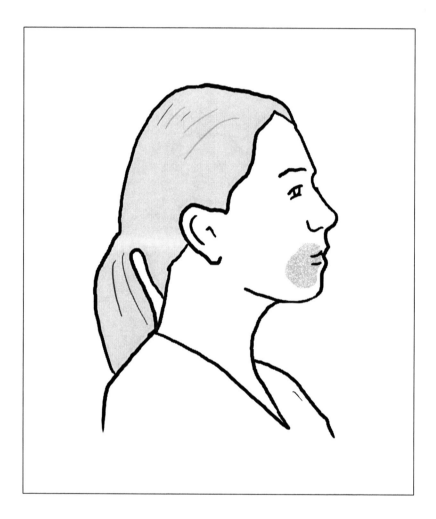

Figure 14-32B: Areas of trigger point relief from the Fish Hook Exercise.

Exercise #30

The Frontalis Exercise

The Frontalis exercise will require great concentration in order to perform correctly. Use all fingers on your hands and place them slightly above your eyebrows and draw the skin upward. Then with great concentration, using the muscles under your fingers, draw your fingers downward. Your eyes will be squinching tighter together as your frontalis muscle pulls your fingertips downward. That is exercising the frontalis and other head muscles of which can contribute to headaches. Perform according to your stage level.

Begin:

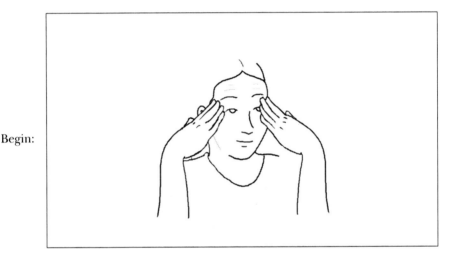

End:

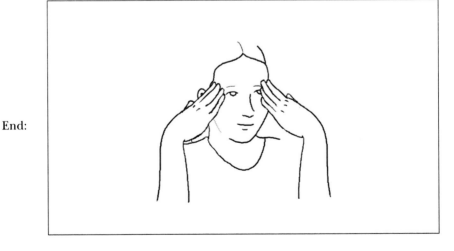

Figure 15-33A: The Frontalis Exercise.

Areas of relief: Frontalis.

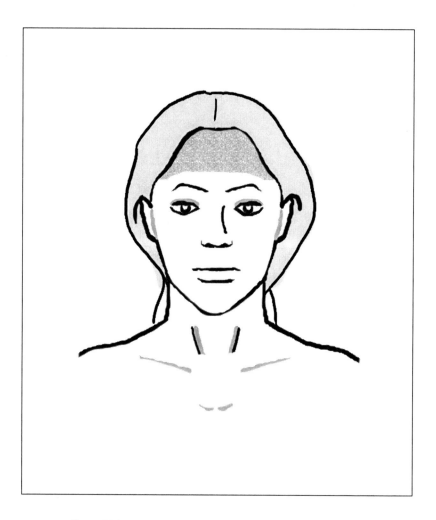

Figure 14-33B: Areas of trigger point relief from the Frontalis Exercise.

Exercise #31

The Occipitalis Exercise

The occipitalis exercise will also help with easing headaches. Again, this exercise will require even greater concentration than the Frontalis exercise. Put your fingertips on the back of your head just a little wide and draw the skin upward. Then, using the muscles on the back of the head draw your fingers downward. It may take a little more concentration than some of the other exercises you've performed. Perform according to your stage level.

Begin:

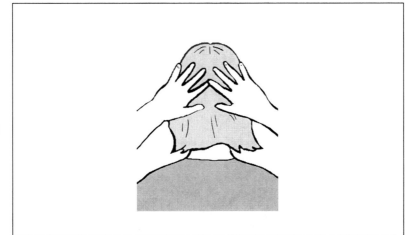

End:

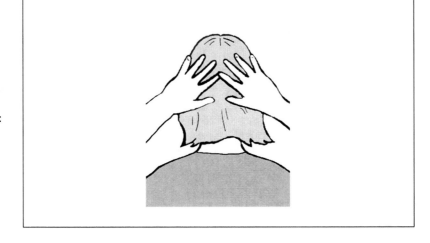

Figure 14-34A: The Occipitalis Exercise.

Areas of relief: Occipitalis

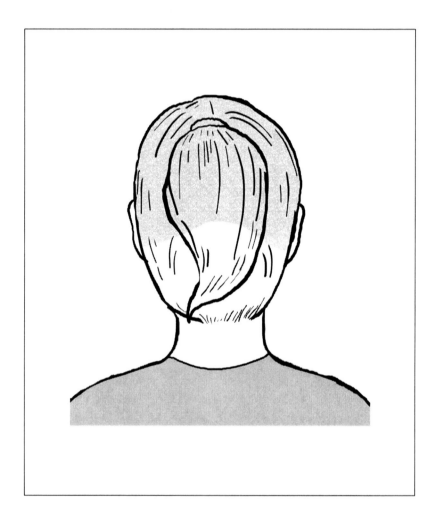

Figure 14-34B: Areas of trigger point relief from the Occipitalis Exercise.

Exercise #32

The Temporalis Exercise

The Temporalis Muscle exercise may be slightly easier to perform than the Frontalis and Occipitalis exercises. Place the palms of your hands slightly above the temples, clasping your fingers together. Pull the skin upward and then using your temporalis muscles, draw them back down. It will work both sides at the same time. Perform according to your stage level, keeping your fingers interlocked.

Begin:

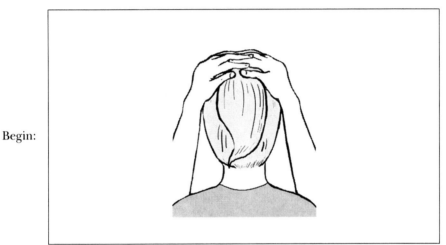

End:

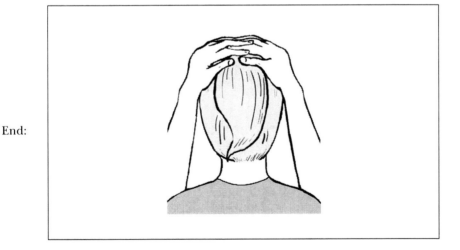

Figure 14-35A: The Temporalis Exercise.

Areas or relief: Temporalis.

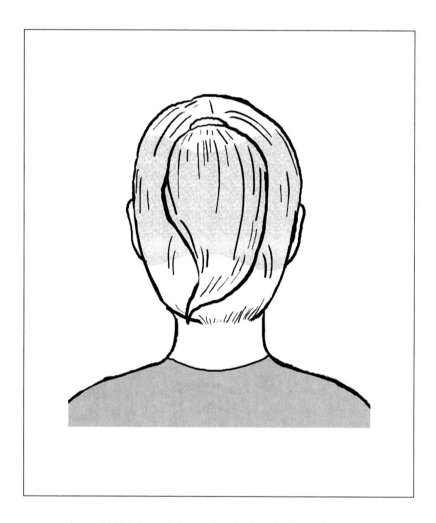

Figure 14-35B: Areas of trigger point relief from the Temporalis Exercise.

Exercise #33

The Advanced Sprint

The Advanced Sprint will help hyperventilation, mitral valve prolapse, tachycardia, heart palpitations, IBS and much more. After your body is in good tone and you have made significant progress, it's time to try to sprint during the middle of your aerobics routine. Whether you are running or cycling makes no difference. Perform it on days you do not lift weights. After sufficiently warming up for about 15 minutes, keep your heart rate up at 70% of your maximum rate, then go ahead and sprint almost as fast as you can and keep it up fast for about 30 seconds. Then, slow down very gradually until you are able to recover your breath very easily. Eventually perform this just 2-4 times on the days you are to perform aerobic exercise only. You only need to do this a couple of times throughout the entire program. Do not perform this on every aerobic workout day.

Important: The Advanced Sprint is an anaerobic exercise for the heart and lungs. So give sufficient time to regain oxygen to the cardiopulmonary system before sprinting again.

This Advanced Sprint can really help with the digestive problems, IBS, constipation and others. Only perform this exercise if you are healthy and in peak shape.

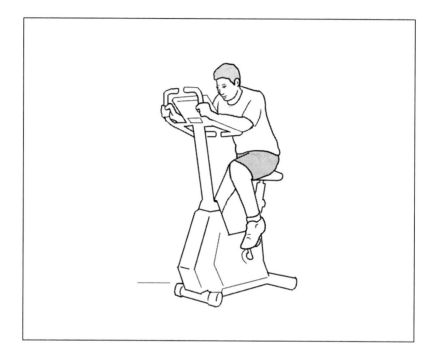

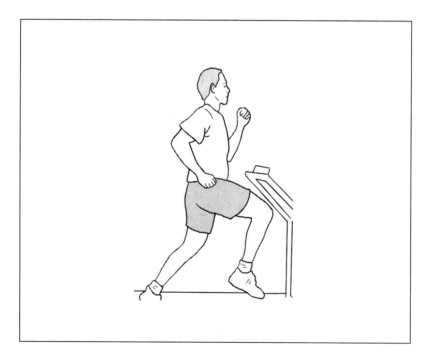

Figure 14-36: The Advanced Sprint.

Areas of relief from the Advanced Sprint: Cardiopulmonary.

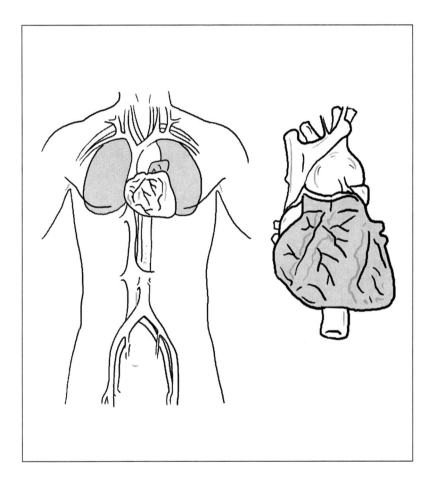

Figure 14-37: The Cardiopulmonary System.

Exercise #34

The Warm Down Exercise

It's time to warm down now. Warm down by performing aerobic exercises for 10-15 minutes. Just like the warm-up, use an aerobic exercise to warm down muscles. At least 10-15 minutes of warm down is sufficient.

Stationary
Bicycle:

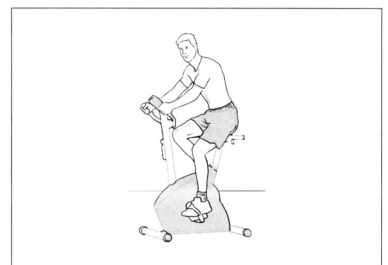

Walk:

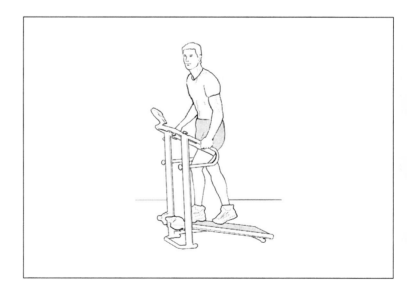

Figure 14-38: The Warm Down.

Sauna Bath

When you are done with your warm down exercises, go to the sauna room for 10 minutes. The benefits of the sauna bath are awesome.

- Helps to burn calories
- Helps to condition heart
- Relieves stress
- Induces deeper sleep
- Relaxes muscles
- Helps to Flush out waste and toxins
- Helps to cleanse the skin
  (various sources)

This is why it is used as a part of the remedy. After warming down and sweating good in the sauna, rest for 15 minutes and then move to the hot tub. This is where you must really let go and let your muscles relax as well for about 10 minutes. You will only need to use the hot tub on the days you actually lift weights, except for additional time you may want to spend in the hot tub to relieve muscle soreness. When the water is at 104° Fahrenheit you will get the best relaxing effect. Although this may be too hot for some, just lower the temperature to your preference. Remember to ease down into the hot water slowly. Be cautious because you don't want it too hot. However, any temperature lower than 104 degrees will not relax you as good. But even 103 degrees is still fairly good. Remember to let the hot tub reach up on your neck muscles as well as the rest of your body.

The hot tub experience

According to a reprinted article from Pool and Spa News (The physiology of Hot water, 2001), a hot tub can be quite a refreshing experience. When you first step into a hot tub you may be taken back with how hot it is, but as the jets propel the water with air combined together it seems quite alright. Smooth sailing, you might say to yourself as you cautiously slip down in. If it wasn't for those jets, my, you wouldn't be able to stand it, so you think. As you get down into the hot water you might feel the sensation of weightlessness as if you were in outer space and then it starts to heat your body up and that's when the pain begins to fade away. Then your heart starts pumping blood at a faster rate in an attempt to cool your body back down. Your blood pressure may increase for a short time and then it will begin to go back down. Your blood goes to the surface of your body and returns to get cooler, similar to that of a radiator. But instead of cooling your body down it encounters the heat from the spa and has no choice but to warm up even more as your blood circulates more and more. The article goes on to say, that your bodies' temperature can be raised up past a 102°

easily in less than 20 minutes. It's like giving yourself a healthy fever as if your body was fighting an infection. A typical thermometer can be used to measure your body temperature as well as the water temperature. As the body heats up, blood vessels begin to dilate, causing easier blood flow so that the cell rate exchange is superiorly enhanced. This dilating of blood vessels is also the cause of the blood pressure dropping. All of this continues to give you the ultimate relaxation experience. Ah, it's almost heaven. As your body gets warmed up deeper and deeper, your muscles begin to relax more and more, taking pressure off of any pinched nerves or blood vessels. It achieves this because it is causing the cell rate exchange to happen more freely and rids your body of wastes. Lactic acid and metabolic waste goes out and your body gets ready for more nutrients to be replenished back again. Lactic acid is found in your blood, muscles, body fluids and organs. But are mostly produced by muscles that obtained energy when oxygen was not present. This is the result of anaerobic exercise. If lactic acid builds up in large amounts it leads to fatigue and can even cause cramps. This is why the hot tub is vitally important for this entire program and not just for pain relief or relaxation. The article continues saying that as these wastes leave, pain leaves. The central nervous system also becomes depressed and this helps muscles relax and relieve tension and pain. While in the hot tub the body starts to break out in a sweat in an attempt to cool down. The pores begin to also open up and release waste as well.

By now, your muscles are completely relaxed and your range of motion is improved which eases off tension and stiffness. Some stretching in the hot tub at this point is not a bad idea either. But not too much. It seems that the jet action in the tub also promotes healing by giving a hydromassage to the area it propels against which in turn can cause the production of endorphins. In addition, the heat and pressure can help to raise the level of antibodies and white blood cells (our little self-induced fever), causing bad cells to be destroyed and stimulating the formation of new ones. This new growth stimulation is one of the goals of this program. And finally, the article says that after you get out of the hot tub your body temperature will begin to fall which is known to cause sleep to deepen. This may help you get that deeper stage IV sleep. Remember to always use moderation and please consult with your physician first (especially if you have a heart condition) before entering any hot tub (The Physiology of Hot water, 2001). After you get the feel of when you are relaxed, then you may shower and return home. If there is no hot tub then take a very warm extended shower or bath (about 10 minutes). Be sure to drink your muscle toning (protein) mix and to eat a healthy meal with it once you arrive home. You will be replenishing the best nutrients available back into your muscle cells by using the protein mix.

Though this regimen seems like it may be difficult at first, you can do it with the help of the CO-Q-10 and the strongest motivation of all, which is that this is a once in a lifetime chance to get out of the constant pain that you've been suffering.

Stretching

Stretching exercises were not a significant part of this program. However, you may want to utilize the following stretches on days you do not perform anaerobic exercises at all. Perform these stretches slowly and easily, while always breathing in a relaxed state and hold them up to 30 seconds each.

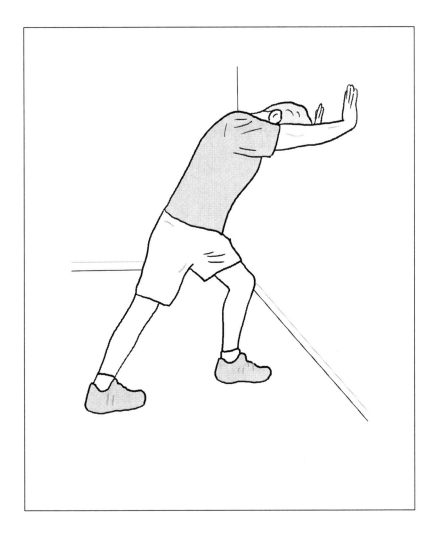

Figure 14-39: The Calf Stretch.

The calves tend to get really tight and stretching them will help relax them. Lean against a wall with one leg behind you keeping rear heel down during the stretch. Move your hips forward toward the wall to feel the calf stretch. Hold for up to 30 seconds then alternate legs.

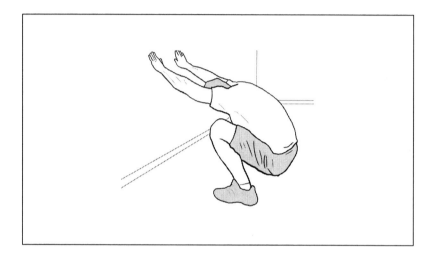

Figure 14-40: The Thigh Stretch.

Slowly squat down while supporting yourself on a wall. The quadriceps should feel the stretch. Stay in this position for up to 30 seconds while breathing in a relaxed manner.

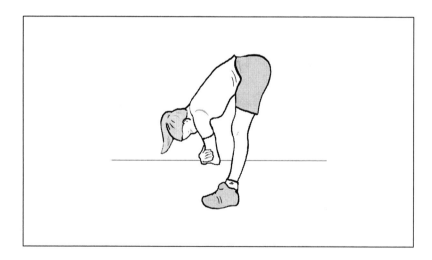

Figure 14-41: The Back Stretch.

With knees partly bent, bend over and reach toward the floor while crossing arms to help stretch the upper back as well as the lower back, hips and hamstrings. Do not strain or force, just relax and breathe. Hold stretch for up to 30 seconds.

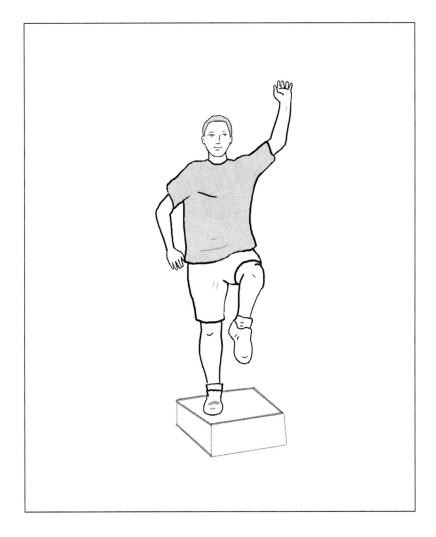

Figure 14-42: The Body Stretch.

Stand and place your right foot on a step and reach your left hand and arm up high. Hold for up to 30 seconds, then alternate.

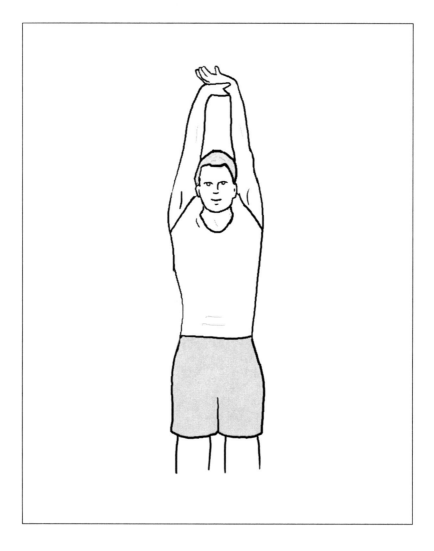

Figure 14-43: The Reach Back Stretch.

In a standing position, reach up and back stretching the front of the chest and the arms. Hold for up to 30 seconds.

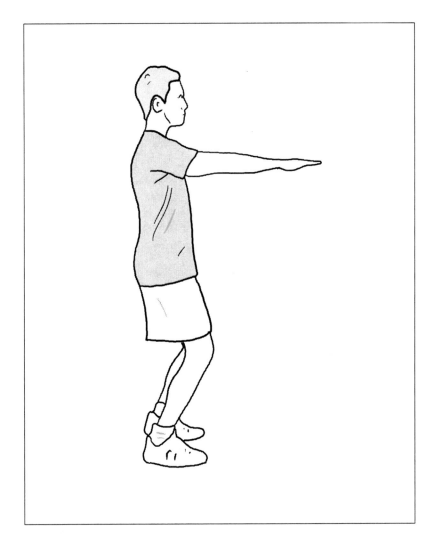

Figure 14-44: The Reach Forward Stretch.

In a standing position, reach your arms forward and stretch for up to 30 seconds.

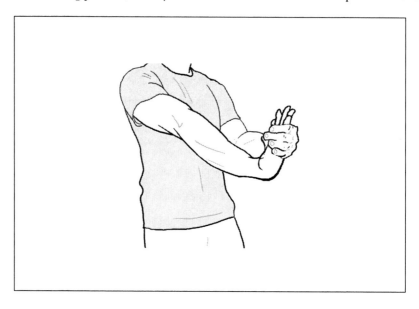

Figure 14-45: The Wrist Flexion.

In a standing position, reach one hand out with the palm facing up. Then, using other hand, hold the fingers and flex your hand downward. Hold for up to 30 seconds, then alternate.

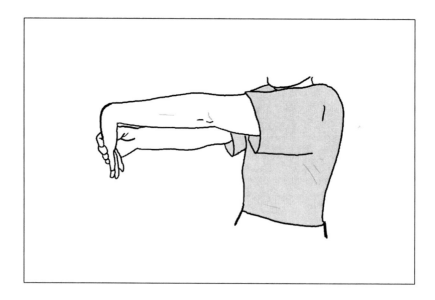

Figure 14-46: The Wrist Extension.

In a standing position, reach one hand out with the palm facing down. Then using other hand hold the back of your hand and extend downward. Hold for up to 30 seconds, then alternate.

Don't overdo it! Regular yawning and the body's natural stretching will be good in helping the body to stretch on its own. Please keep stretching to a minimum. You don't want to overstretch because overstretching will make joints become hypermobile and that will not work to your advantage as FMS, MPS, CFS and GWS affect joints in a negative and painful way. These are all of the exercises required to get the desired results that you're looking for.

For your convenience there is a complete workout list in the proper chronological order contained in Appendix B. You can keep records of the amount of weight that you use on this workout list.

PART III

THE RECOVERY

CHAPTER 15

What Is A Miracle?

When people think of miracles, they may think of the birth of a baby or someone surviving getting struck by lightning or even the Shroud of Turin. These may qualify very well but what about you getting a specific answer to your prayer for your specific need? Especially when that same answer doesn't happen to others on a regular basis. Would you be impressed then? What if you get an answer to your prayer for you to be healed of your illness or at least the symptoms that go with it? Would that be considered a miracle to you? Especially when seeing that not many at all can have that type of testimony. Have you ever sincerely prayed to God that you would get better? Or is it just wishful hoping or thinking? Miracles belong to God and his people; however he does heal Gentiles (unsaved) folks of diseases and illnesses like he did for Naaman. Let's read that story in II Kings 5:1-19, "Now Naaman, captain of the host of the king of Syria, was a great man with his master, and honourable, because by him the Lord had given deliverance unto Syria; he was also a mighty man in valour, but he was a leper. And the Syrians had gone out by companies, and had brought away captive out of the land of Israel a little maid; and she waited on Naaman's wife. And she said unto her mistress, Would God my lord were with the prophet that is in Samaria! for he would recover him of his leprosy. And one went in, and told his lord, saying, Thus and thus said the maid that is of the land of Israel. And the king of Syria said, Go to, go, and I will send a letter unto the king of Israel. And he departed, and took with him ten talents of silver, and six thousand pieces of gold, and ten changes of raiment. And he brought the letter to the king of Israel, saying, Now when this letter is come unto thee, behold, I have therewith sent Naaman my servant to thee, that thou mayest recover him of his leprosy. And it came to pass, when the king of Israel had read the letter, that he rent his clothes, and said, Am I God, to kill and to make alive, that this man doth send unto me to recover a man of his leprosy? wherefore consider, I pray you, and see how he seeketh a quarrel against me. And it was so, when Elisha the man of God had heard that the king of Israel had rent his clothes, that he sent to the king, saying, Wherefore hast thou rent thy clothes? let him come now to me, and he shall know that there is a prophet in Israel. So Naaman came with his horses and with his chariot, and stood at the door of the house of Elisha. And Elisha sent a messenger unto him, saying, Go and wash in Jordan seven times, and thy flesh shall come again to thee, and thou shalt be clean. But Naaman was wroth, and went away, and said, Behold, I thought, He will surely come out to me, and stand, and call on the name of the Lord his God, and strike his hand over the place, and recover the leper. Are not Abana and Pharpar, rivers of Damascus, better than all the waters of Israel? may I not wash in them, and be clean? So he turned and went away in a rage. And his servants came near, and spake unto him, and said, My father, if the prophet had bid thee do some great thing, wouldest thou not have done it? how much rather then, when he saith to thee, Wash, and be clean? Then he went down, and dipped himself seven times in Jordan, according to the saying of the man of God: and his flesh came again like unto the flesh of a little child, and he was clean. And he returned to the man of God, he and all his company, and came, and stood before him: and he said, Behold, now I know that there is no God in all the earth, but in Israel: now therefore, I pray thee, take a blessing of thy servant. But he said, As the Lord liveth, before whom I stand, I will receive none. And he urged him to take it; but he refused. And Naaman said, Shall there not then, I pray thee, be given to thy servant two mules' burden of earth? for thy servant will henceforth offer neither burnt offering nor sacrifice unto other gods, but unto the Lord. In this thing the Lord pardon thy servant, that when my master goeth into the house of Rimmon to worship there, and he leaneth on my hand, and I bow down myself in the house of Rimmon, the Lord pardon thy servant in this thing. And he said unto him, Go in peace. So he departed from him a little way." Naaman was from Syria (Gentile nation). It was his little maid (Jew) who was taken captive from Israel that encouraged him to see a man of God back in Samaria. That man of God was Elisha. He's a prophet, a preacher, a Jew, a believer, one who keeps the oracles of God. It was this type of man God chose to work through. In like manner if God chose me to tell you to perform this program for up to 8 weeks and you'd get your healing, isn't that just like how Elisha told Naaman to dip in the Jordan River seven times to get his healing? So if your problem goes away, should you claim it as a miracle? If not, why not? You must remember that the Jordan River was always there even before Elisha or Naaman were born. Many people went and used the river to bathe in and later to get baptized in. John the Baptist, Jesus Christ, and many others were baptized in the Jordan River. The Jordan River was even halted at one time when Israel passed over it to take the land of Canaan. God used someone with leprosy (an illness), a dirty river (the Jordan) and a man of God (the prophet Elisha) to get results for just one miracle. So why didn't all the lepers just go dip seven times in the Jordan River like Naaman to get their healing? This is where the supernatural power of God and his divine timing makes the world stand back in awe. In the same manner, why didn't scientists discover the same remedy that I have before me? Because of divine timing friend. That's why.

> *This New Breakthrough is a true and great miracle from God.*
>
> R.D.G.

Some may define a miracle as an event or occurrence of which it is a rare thing to happen whether going against the laws of nature or not. If it is rare enough then it just may be considered a miracle. Some of these events or occurrences might even be classified as signs, wonders or powers. It could even be an act of compassion by the Lord our God to heal someone of something that's not otherwise easy to be healed of.

Why do miracles happen? We know that they happen to manifest the works of God so that others might know the power and sovereignty of God. There is only one God and there is none like him in neither heaven nor earth.

In Mark 2:3-12 it reads: "And they come unto him, bringing one sick of the palsy, which was borne of four. And when they could not come nigh unto him for the press, they uncovered the roof where he was: and when they had broken it up, they let down the bed wherein the sick of the palsy lay. When Jesus saw their faith, he said unto the sick of the palsy, Son, thy sins be forgiven thee. But there were certain of the scribes sitting there, and reasoning in their hearts, Why doth this man thus speak blasphemies? who can forgive sins but God only? And immediately when Jesus perceived in his spirit that they so reasoned within themselves, he said unto them, Why reason ye these things in your hearts? Whether is it easier to say to the sick of the palsy, Thy sins be forgiven thee; or to say, Arise, and take up thy bed, and walk? But that ye may know that the Son of man hath power on earth to forgive sins, (he saith to the sick of the palsy,) I say unto thee, Arise, and take up thy bed, and go thy way into thine house. And immediately he arose, took up the bed, and went forth before them all; insomuch that they were all amazed, and glorified God saying, We never saw it on this fashion."

This was quite a miracle for a paralytic man. I want you to notice in vs.5 that Jesus Christ looked on the others' faith and not just the sick one with palsy. This is a great lesson. In addition to that the religious crowd was thinking evil against Jesus Christ for the power that he had which is not only healing the sick of the palsy but forgiving him of his sins. Salvation and healing go hand in hand.

We also see that healing and salvation go hand in hand in James 5:14-15. "Is any sick among you? Let him call for the elders (ministers) of the church; and let them pray over him, anointing him with oil in the name of the Lord: And the prayer of faith shall save the sick, and the Lord shall raise him up; and if he hath committed sins, they shall be forgiven him."

I've even did this many times prior to having my healing manifested. It's only the right thing to do.

Another miracle that the Lord had performed is found in Luke 13:11-17. "And, behold, there was a woman which had a spirit of infirmity eighteen years, and was bowed together, and could in no wise lift up herself. And when Jesus saw her, he called her to him, and said unto her, Woman, thou art loosed from thine infirmity. And he laid his hands on her; and immediately she was made straight, and glorified God. And the ruler of the synagogue answered with indignation, because that Jesus had healed on the sabbath day, and said unto the people, There are six days in which men ought to work: in them therefore come and be healed, and not on the sabbath day. The Lord then answered him, and said, Thou hypocrite, doth not each one of you on the Sabbath loose his ox or his ass from the stall, and lead him away to watering? And ought not this woman, being a daughter of Abraham, whom Satan hath bound, lo, these eighteen years, be loosed from this bond on the Sabbath day? And when he had said these things, all his adversaries were ashamed; and all the people rejoiced for all the glorious things that were done by him." This woman had a chronic ailment and yet she was able to be loosed of it after 18 years. That's encouraging. Once again the religious folks found fault with the Lord for healing on the Sabbath day. He says in Mark 2: 27-28, "And he said unto them, The Sabbath was made for man, and not man for the Sabbath: Therefore the Son of man is Lord also of the Sabbath."

One miracle for me was when my wife found that I no longer had trigger points all over my body. And even more than that was when my Rheumatologist also checked me all over my body and confirmed that I definitely no longer had trigger points or tender points whatsoever. Those two together were some of the highest points in my life ever since I was diagnosed with FMS, MPS, CFS and AA. I still remember back in 1991 the massages that I had to have everyday by my wife and the massages by the therapist for my condition. The anesthesiologist would inject my muscles with corticosteroids all over my neck, shoulders and back trying to get rid of or break up the myofoscial trigger points. After the injections, there was the ultrasound over these injected areas. I was even placed on a traction machine several times to no avail. But lastly there was that massage therapist. And she really worked out the trigger points using her thumbs, fingers and even her elbows. That used to give some relief but within a day or so they'd be back along with all of the pain. In 1996, I found out through my wife's check ups for trigger points and tender points that I was healed but I still went to the Doctor (a Rheumatologist) to get my healing confirmed. I still remember that appointment because I had taken my brother with me as a witness. I had to strip down to nothing but my underwear (routine for this type of check up). The doctor returned back to the room with my brother present as a witness and he proceeded to check my ankles, calves, thighs, arms, back, shoulders, neck and abdomen and he could not find one tender point or trigger point on my entire body. You should've seen the look on his face when he asked, "What did you do?" He was awe-struck.

I need to stress a point about miracles and healing. Healing usually takes place over a period of time and is not instantaneous like that of a miracle. Yet even though people get healed over the process of time, they still do refer to their healing as a miracle, I do. When people get ill and/or disabled most of the time they just want the world to stop and stand still for them. And that can sometimes leave people in a sense of despair. Almost every time this happens we can see that the Devil has stolen some good things from these people. Good things like:

- Praise
- The Joy of Your Salvation
- Hope
- Sense of Well Being
- Happiness, etc . . .

The Devil will try to get you to believe the fearful thoughts again and again but you need to rebuke and revenge those thoughts. II Corinthians 10:3-6 says, "For though we walk in the flesh, we do not war after the flesh: (For the weapons of our warfare are not carnal, but mighty through God to the pulling down of strong holds;) Casting down imaginations, and every high thing that exalteth itself against the knowledge of God, and bringing into captivity every thought to the obedience of Christ; And having in a readiness to revenge all disobedience, when your obedience is fulfilled."

Many times we go through hardships that may seem like we're not able to bear. But God promised us he wouldn't put on us more than we could bear. In I Corinthians 10:13 it reads, "There hath no temptation taken you but such as is common to man: but God is faithful, who will not suffer you to be tempted above that ye are able; but will with the temptation also make a way to escape, that ye may be able to bear it." The Lord also says seek me while you are young, while it is early and in Jeremiah 29:13 it says, "And ye shall seek me, and find me, when ye shall search for me with all your heart." If you don't have faith you'll never take the steps needed to bridge the gap between where you are and where you desire to be. It takes faith. He promised us healing and he also promised us in Ephesians 3:20-21, "Now unto him that is able to do exceeding abundantly above all that we ask or think, according to the power that worketh in us, Unto him be glory in the church by Christ Jesus throughout all ages, world without end. Amen." And it's this area that one must tap into to see the true riches of God and to receive the inheritance that he has for his children. For it says in Luke 12:32 "Fear not, little flock; for it is your Father's good pleasure to give you the kingdom." If we are not faithful in unrighteous mammon, who will entrust us with the true riches from heaven? These are the true riches I'm talking about, an inheritance from God, something we don't work for but is a free gift simply because we are related to the King of kings and Lord of lords. He's able to give his riches to his children. I'll repeat III John 2 again, "Beloved, I wish above all things that thou mayest prosper and be in health, even as thy soul prospereth."

If you want healing you are going to have to exercise your faith in God and look for the answer.

Will you lay back in loss of hope, anger, disappointment or will you rejoice that God has done something wonderful in your life through healing your sickly body, through making you well again. In all of these situations God is still able to heal anybody of anything. In Philippians 4:4-7; it reads: "Rejoice in the Lord alway: and again I say, Rejoice. Let your moderation be known unto all men. The Lord is at hand. Be careful for nothing; but in every thing by prayer and supplication with thanksgiving let your requests be made known unto God. And the peace of God, which passeth all understanding, shall keep your hearts and minds through Christ Jesus." So the big question to you is will you exercise your faith? In Hebrews 11:6 it says, "But without faith it is impossible to please him: for he that cometh to God must believe that he is, and that he is a rewarder of them that diligently seek him." If Naaman and the others could be healed then you can get your healing too. God's not a respecter of persons. When the angel of the Lord told Abraham that his wife, Sarah, was going to have a child in her old age, she laughed in unbelief, but the angel confronted her with the question, "Is anything too hard for the Lord?"

The greatest lesson we've just learned is that in order to get a miracle, you've got to be expecting a miracle. If you want healing you are going to have to exercise your faith in God and look for the answer. Don't settle for anything less than what you are hoping, praying, expecting and believing for.

CHAPTER 16

Rehabilitation

The remedy in this program can restore almost everything you lost due to FMS, MPS, CFS, CFIDS, GWS and Anxiety Attacks. But what kind of work are you going to be able to perform if you are able to perform any at all? You'll be more than ready health wise but now what else can you do or train for that will not knock you out of productivity or from being gainfully employed altogether again? Prior to moving on to employment, first try taking care of your own personal business by using this simple outline of your everyday workload (see list).

Workload

- Bath and Hygiene—clip nails, floss, cut hair
- Appointments
- Phone Calls, E-mail, Faxing
- Mail—get mail, mail out, file rack
- Notebook—main, current list
- Shop
- Cook, Wash Dishes, Clean Microwave
- Wash clothes
- Clean, garbage, dust, cobwebs, spray for bugs, bathroom, sweep, mop
- Straighten up
- Mow lawn, rake leaves, shovel snow, salt sidewalk, herbicide
- Exercise
- Car maintenance
- Check off budget, bills, checkbook, call bank
- Pick up cleaners, shirts
- Back Burner
- Refill meds
- End of month Accounting—gather all receipts
- B-day & cards, calendar events
- File stuff

- Follow-ups
- Other

After sufficient progress is made from your personal workload list, you may be able to add some more good stress onto your workload. You may be able to resume your old employment fairly well while others may need schooling and/or vocational rehabilitation services. There is a vocational rehabilitation office in every state throughout the United States. Foreigners may check with their country for similar services.

The following list can help you choose a career of your choice, but is actually meant to refresh your memory of all of the possibilities that are out there for you. So try to choose a job that won't be too hard to perform since you have been afflicted with one or more of these syndromes. Hopefully many patients will be able to return back to some type of employment and help to restore those things that they've lost as a result of these conditions. For it says in Joel 2:25-26, "And I will restore to you the years that the locust hath eaten, the cankerworm, and the caterpillar, and the palmerworm, my great army which I sent among you. And ye shall eat in plenty, and be satisfied, and praise the name of the Lord your God, that hath dealt wondrously with you: and my people shall never be ashamed" (See list).

Accountant
Actor
Actuary
Advertising Account Executive
Advertising Manager
Advertising Salesperson
Advertising Worker
Aerospace Engineer
Air-conditioning, Refrigeration and Heating Technician
Airplane Mechanic
Airplane Pilot
Airport Manager
Air Traffic Controller
Appliance Repairer
Architect
Athlete, Professional
Athletic Coach
Automotive Mechanic
Bank Officer
Bank Teller
Boichemist
Biomedical Engineer

Broadcast Technician
Building Contractor
Building or Property Manager
Business Machine Service Technician
Carpenter
Cartoonist
Ceramic Engineer
Chef
Chemical Engineer
Chemist
Childcare Worker
Chiropractor
City Manager
Civil Engineer
Claim Representative
Communications Equipment Mechanic
Computer Programmer
Computer Service Technician
Controller
Corrections Officer
Cosmetologist
Credit Investigator
Credit Manager
Criminologist
Dancer
Dental Assistant
Dental Hygienist
Dentist
Dietician
Drafter
Economist
Editor, Book Publishing
Editor, Newspaper and Magazine
Electrical/Electronics Engineer
Electrician
Emergency Medical Technician
Employment Counselor
Engineer
Environmentalist
Farmer
Fashion Designer
Forester

Forestry Technician
Funeral Director
Geographer
Geologist
Geophysicist
Graphic Designer
Guard
Guidance Counselor
Health Services Manager
Historian
Home Economist
Hotel/Motel Manager
Industrial Designer
Industrial Engineer
Insurance Agent and Broker
Interior Designer
Interpreter
Investment Manager
Janitor
Labor Relations Specialist
Landscape Architect
Lawyer
Librarian
Life Scientist
Lobbyist
Machinist
Management Consultant
Manufacturer's Sales Representative
Market Analyst
Marketing Manager
Marketing Researcher
Mathematician
Mechanical Engineer
Medical Assistant
Medical Laboratory Technologist
Medical Record Technician
Medical Secretary
Metallurgical Engineer
Meteorologist
Mining Engineer
Minister
Model

Museum Curator
Musician
Newspaper Reporter
Nurse, Licensed Practical
Nurse, Registered
Nursery Worker
Occupational Therapist
Oceanographer
Office Manager
Officer, U.S. Armed Forces
Operating Engineer
Operations Research Analyst
Opthalmologist
Optician, Dispensing
Optometrist
Osteopathic Physician
Paralegal
Parole Officer
Personnel Manager
Petroleum Engineer
Pharmacist
Photographer
Photographic Laboratory Technician
Physical Therapist
Physician
Physician Assistant
Physicist
Plumber and Pipefitter
Podiatrist
Police Officer, Municipal
Police Officer, State
Priest
Printing Press Operator
Producer/Director of Radio, Television, Movies, and Theater
Production Manager, Industrial
Psychiatrist
Psychologist
Public Relations Worker
Purchasing Agent
Rabbi
Radio/Television Announcer
Radiological (X-Ray) Technologist

Range Manager
Real Estate Agent/Broker
Real Estate Appraiser
Recreation Worker
Rehabilitation Counselor
Respiratory Therapist
Retail Buyer
Retail Sales Worker
Retail Store Manager
Safety Engineer
Sales Manager
School Administrator
Secret Service Agent
Secretary
Securities Sales Worker (Stockbroker)
Singer
Social Worker
Sociologist
Soil Conservationist
Soil Scientist
Speech Pathologist and Audiologist
Statistician
Surveyor
Systems Analyst
Teacher, College and University
Teacher, Kindergarten and Elementary School
Teacher, Secondary School
Technical Writer
Television and Radio Service Technician
Tool-and-Die Maker
Traffic Manager, Industrial
Translator
Travel Agent
Truck Driver
Underwriter
Urban Planner
Veterinarian
Waiter
Wholesaler
Word Processor
(Reprinted with permission from VGM, 1997)

To find the nearest vocational rehabilitation office nearest you call 1+ (area code) +555-1212 and ask for your state's vocational rehabilitation office. It's that easy. You may also want to contact a private vocational counselor near you for a second opinion. Private vocational counselors seem to have your interest more at heart. Here are other places to get more information and help:

Guaranteed Student Loans
(Guaranteed Student Loans—84.032)
Federal Student Aid Information Center
P.O. Box 84
Washington, D.C. 20044   800-433-3248
To authorize guaranteed loans for educational expenses available from eligible lenders such as banks, credit unions, savings and loan associations, pension funds, insurance companies, and schools to vocational, undergraduate, and graduate students enrolled at all eligible postsecondary institutions. Estimate of annual funds available: $19,961,182,000.

Get Loans Directly from Your School
(Federal Direct Student Loan Program—number to be announced)
Federal Student Aid Information Center
P.O. Box 84
Washington, D.C. 20044   800-433-3248
To provide loans directly to students through schools, rather than through private lenders. Direct lending will save taxpayers an estimated $4.8 billion dollars, and make borrowing simpler, faster and easier. Estimate of annual funds available: N/A.

Work-Study Programs to Pay for School
(Federal Work-Study Program—84.033)
Federal Student Aid Information Center
P.O Box 84
Washington, DC   800-433-3248
To provide part-time employment to eligible postsecondary students to help meet educational expenses and encourage students receiving program assistance to participate in community service activities. Estimate of annual funds available: $526,941,000

Grants to Study Library Science
(Library Education and Human Resource Development—84.036)
Discretionary Library Programs Division
Library Programs
Office of Educational Research and Improvement
U.S. Department of Education
555 New Jersey Ave., NW, Room 300
Washington, DC 20208   202-219-1315
To assist institutions of higher education and library organizations and agencies in training or retraining persons in areas of library specialization where there are shortages, in new techniques of information acquisition, transfer and communication technology; in library leadership through advanced training in library management, in library education, in advanced training in management of new organizational formats (networks, consortia, etc.), and in serving the information needs of the elderly, the illiterate, disadvantaged or rural residents. Estimate of annual funds available: $4,960,000.

Low-Interest Student Loans
(Federal Perkins Loan Program—Federal Capital Contributions—84.038)
Federal Student Aid Information Center
P.O. Box 84
Washington, DC 20044   800-433-3248
To provide low-interest loans to eligible postsecondary students with demonstrated financial need to help meet educational expenses. Estimate of annual funds available: $144,037,000.

Get Help to Study
(Upward Bound—84.047)
Division of Student Services
Education Outreach Branch
Office of Postsecondary Education
U.S. Department of Education
600 Independent Ave., SW
Portals Bldg., Suite 600D
Washington, DC 20202   202-708-4804
To generate skills and motivation necessary for success in education beyond high school among low-income and potential first-generation college students and veterans. The goal of the program is to increase the academic performance and motivational levels of eligible enrollees so that they have a better chance of completing secondary school and successfully pursuing postsecondary educational programs. Estimate of annual funds available: Grants: $145,938,000; Math/Science Regional Centers: $14,600,000.

$2,300 Grants to Go to School
(Federal Pell Grant Program—84.063)
Division of Policy Development
Student Financial Assistance Programs
Office of Postsecondary Education
U.S. Department of Education
600 Independence Ave., S.W.
Washington, DC 20202   202-708-4607
To provide eligible undergraduate postsecondary students who have demonstrated financial need with grant assistance in meeting educational expenses. Estimate of annual funds available: $6,096,087,000.

$5,000 from Your State to Go to College
(Grants to States for State Student Incentives—84.069)
Division of Policy Development
Student Financial Assistance Programs
Office of Postsecondary Education
U.S. Department of Education
600 Independence Ave, S.W.
Washington, DC 20202   202-708-4607
To provide grants to the States for use in programs that provides financial assistance to eligible postsecondary students. Estimate of annual funds available: $72,555,000.

Grants to Graduate Students
(Patricia Roberts Harris Fellowships—84.094)
Cosette Ryan
Division of Higher Education Incentive Programs
Office of Postsecondary Education
U.S. Department of Education
600 Independence Ave, S.W.
Washington, DC 20202   202-260-3608
In order to help students achieve the master's level, professional, or doctoral education, grants are given to colleges and universities to fund fellowships, particularly for women and members of minority groups who are obtaining degrees in fields of high national priority. Estimate of annual funds available: $21,796,000.

Experimental Job Training Opportunities
Office of Strategic Planning and Policy Development
Employment and Training Administration
U.S. Department of Labor
200 Constitution Ave., NW, Room N5637
Washington, DC 20210   202-219-7674, x153
This office plans and implements Pilot and Demonstration Programs to provide job training, employment opportunities, and related services for individuals with specific disadvantages. These programs address industry-wide skill shortages and offer technical expertise to particular client groups. They also develop information networks among organizations with similar Job Training Partnership Act-related objectives. Administered at the National level and operated at the state and local level, these programs cover disadvantaged groups in the labor market, including offenders, individuals with limited English language proficiency, handicapped person, women, single parents, displaced homemakers, youth, older workers, those who lack educational credentials and public assistance recipients.

Highly Skilled Jobs Apprenticeship
Bureau of Apprenticeship and Training
Employment and Training Administration
U.S. Department of Labor
200 Constitution Ave., NW, Room N4649
Washington, DC 20210   202-219-5540
Apprenticeship is a combination of on-the-job training and related classroom instruction in which workers learn the practical and theoretical aspects of a highly skilled occupation. Apprenticeship programs are operated on a voluntary basis by employers, employer associations, or management and labor groups. The role of the federal government is to encourage and promote the establishment of apprenticeship programs and provide technical assistance to program sponsors. The related classroom instruction is given in the program sponsor's training facility or a local technical school or junior college.

Future Job Trends by Occupation
Superintendent of Documents
Government Printing Office   202-512-1800
Washington, DC 20402   Fax: 202-512-2250
A supplement to the latest edition of the *Occupational Outlook Handbook, Occupational Projections and Training Data* provides detailed, comprehensive statistics and technical data supporting the information presented in the *Handbook*. It also presents a broad overview of expected trends in employment in the mid 1990's and provides employment data for approximately 250 occupations profiled in the *Handbook*. This

supplement is a key reference source for training officials, education planners, and vocational and employment counselors. The cost is $5.50, SN #029-001-03189-1.

Health Professions and Training Programs
Division of Public Health Professions
Health Resources and Services Administration
5600 Fishers Lane, Room 8-101
Rockville, MD 20857   301-443-6854
This division supports programs and provides grants for the following areas: Geriatric Education Centers; Rural Areas Health Care; Dentistry; Schools of Public Health; Preventive Medicine Residency Training; and Graduate Programs in Health Administration. Call for more information on programs.

Information and Records Management Training
Records Administration Information Center
National Archives and Records Administration
8601 Adelphi Rd., Room 2200, Mail Stop NI
College Park, MD 20740-6001   301-713-6677
The Directory of Records Administration Training Programs in the Washington, DC Area lists classes available from government, academic, and private sources in such subject areas as records management, Information Resource Management, micrographics and optical disks. Basic courses currently being offered include: Introduction to Records Management; Files Improvement; and Records Disposition. Contact this office for a copy.

International Trade Commission Jobs
Office of Personnel
U.S. International Trade Commission
500 E. St., SW, Room 314
Washington, DC 20436   202-205-2651
Information on employment can be obtained from the Personnel Director. Personnel employed include international economists, attorneys, accountants, commodity and industry specialists and analysts, and clerical and other support personnel.

Job Corps Conservation Centers
Office of Historically Black College and University Programs and Job Corps
U.S. Department of the Interior
18th and C Sts., NW

Job Corps for Youths
Office of Job Corps
Employment and Training Administration
U.S. Department of Labor
200 Constitution Ave., NW 800-733-JOBS
Washington, DC 20001   202-219-8550
The Job Corps, a Federally administered national employment and training program, is designed to serve severely disadvantaged youth 16-21 years old. Enrollees are provided food, housing, education, vocational training, medical care, counseling, and other support services. The program prepares youth for stable, productive employment and entrance into vocational/technical schools or other institutions for further education or training. Job Corps centers range in capacity from 175 to 2,600 enrollees. Some of the centers are operated by the U.S. Departments of Interior and Agriculture (civilian conservation centers), while the remaining centers are operated under contracts with the U.S. Department of Labor primarily by major corporations. Vocational training is given in such occupations as auto repair, carpentry, painting, nursing, business and clerical skills, as well as preparation for the General Education Development high school equivalency examination. To apply, contact a Job Service office, or call the Job Corps Alumni Association's toll-free number: 800-424-2866.

Jobs for Seniors 55 Years and Up
Office of Special Targeted Programs
Employment and Training Administration
U.S. Department of Labor
200 Constitution Ave., NW, Room N4643   202-219-5904
Washington, DC 20210   TDD: 800-326-2577
Sponsored by state and territorial governments and ten national organizations, the Senior Community Service Employment Program (SCSEP) promotes the creation of part-time jobs in community service activities for jobless, low-income persons who are at least 55 years of age and have poor employment prospects. Individuals work in part-time jobs at senior citizens centers, in schools or hospitals, in programs for the handicapped, in fire prevention programs, and on beautification and restoration projects. This program makes possible and array of community services to the elderly. SCSEP participants must be at least 55 years of age, have family income of not more than 25% above the Federal poverty level, and be capable of performing the tasks to which they are assigned. For more information, contact state offices for the aging, area agencies on aging, local job service offices, or this office.

Job Training and Employment Publications

Superintendent of Documents
Government Printing Office   202-512-1800
Washington, DC 20402   Fax: 202-512-2250

The Government Printing Office (GPO) sells hundreds of publications on employment and occupations. Call GPO and ask for Subject Bibliographies 044 and 202, which contain lists of available publications and their prices. The Subject Bibliographies are free. You can have these documents faxed to you by using GPO Faxwatch at 202-512-1716

Job Training and Employment Services

Office of the Assistant Secretary for Employment and Training
U.S. Department of Labor
200 Constitution Ave, NW, Room S2321
Washington, DC 20210   202-219-6050

The Job Training Partnership Act provides job training and employment services for economically disadvantaged adults and youth, dislocated workers, and others who face significant employment barriers. The goal of this Act is to move the jobless into permanent, unsubsidized, self-sustaining employment. State and local governments have primary responsibility for the management and administration of job training programs. In addition, a new public/private partnership has been created to plan and design training programs as well as to deliver training and other services.

Job Training and Workplace Research and Development

Office of Strategic Planning and Policy Development
Employment and Training Administration
U.S. Department of Labor
200 Constitution Ave., NW, Room N5637
Washington, DC 20210   202-219-7674, x153

Research, Demonstration, and Evaluation Projects summarizes the projects funded by the Employment and Training Administration. The most recent focus has been on workplace literacy, youth, worker adjustment, women-families-welfare, and improving employment and training programs. This free catalog provides several indexes and ordering information.

Local Help for Job Seekers
Employment and Training Administration
U.S. Department of Labor
200 Constitution Ave., NW, Room N4470
Washington, DC 20210   202-219-5257
The U.S. Employment Service, through affiliated state employment agencies, operates almost 2,000 local employment service (job service) offices. They assist job seekers in finding employment and assist employers in filling job vacancies. They administer occupational aptitude tests and circulate information about jobs and training opportunities.

Matching Yourself with the Workworld
Superintendent of Documents
Government Printing Office   202-512-1800
Washington, DC 20402   Fax: 202-512-2250
Designed to assist you in comparing job characteristics with your skills and interests, the publication, *Matching Yourself with the World of Work,* lists and defines 17 occupational characteristics and requirements, and matches these characteristics with 200 occupations chosen from the 1988-89 *Occupational Outlook Handbook* It is available for $1, SN #029-001-02910-1.

Job Retraining for Free
Get free technical and vocational training under a federal job-training program through your local employment office.

Jobs With the Federal Government
Most federal agencies have job line recordings for immediate openings that need filling. Consult the U.S. Government listings in your phone book for the appropriate agency and number, or see the chapter on Federal Government Databases for the listings in Washington, DC headquarters.

Job Trends: What's Hot, What's Not
Office of Employment Projectors
U.S. Department of Labor
2 Massachusetts Avenue, NE, Room 2135
Washington, DC 20212   202-606-5709
Find out what jobs will be hot and what will not before you spend money on college.

When searching for vocational rehabilitation services or other options, be sure to take in consideration some of the following possible residual problems associated with your newfound health. Some believe that this program is a total cure for Myofascial Pain Syndrome while yet leaving some residual problems from Fibromyalgia or Chronic Fatigue Syndrome. Just getting out of constant pain is a great big prayer answered. So, are there any residual problems? From time to time you may feel a little fatigue but what's that compared to years of feeling extremely fatigued? Certainly you've handled worse before and even worse still is that it will go on for your whole lifetime if you never take action to complete this comprehensive program. Sometimes you may even feel slightly stiff in the morning but it's not like before and soon you'll have forgotten what it was like to feel stiff in the morning. Just wait and see. The morning stiffness has about diminished to the point of not being present. However, the non-restorative stage IV sleep continues to be a slight residual problem. But it has still improved considerably. Memory has improved to a tolerable level. The so-called fibrofog is also diminished to null as well. The panic attacks have just about totally dissipated. However, the sleep problem and fatigue should be minimized at the plateau of your wellness. It should also stay better throughout the rest of your life.

Once in a while there is still some muscle twitching but it's tolerable because there is no pain associated with it. The tender points, trigger points and constant widespread musculoskeletal pain have been permanently removed from your body, unless of course you get another illness or injury that could trigger some of these signs and symptoms again. If you'd like to measure your degree of healing, use the following list to compare what you are like before this program and then take the test again to look at the dramatic improvement in your health afterwards. I'm sure you will agree that it's truly a miracle. (See list).

Identify all of your symptoms:

_____ Multiple tender points	_____ Numbness and tingling
_____ Nonrestorative sleep	_____ Sicca symptoms
_____ Chronic fatigue	_____ Raynaud's phenomenon
_____ Morning stiffness	_____ Dysmenorrhea
_____ Subjective swelling	_____ Anxiety
_____ Irritable Bowel Syndrome	_____ Panic attacks
_____ Depression	_____ Frequent severe headaches
_____ Mitral valve prolapse	_____ Female urethral syndrome
_____ Hypothyroidism	_____ Premenstrual syndrome
_____ Vestibular dysfunction	_____ Carpal tunnel syndrome
_____ Incoordination	_____ Chronic fatigue syndrome
_____ Cognitive impairment	_____ TMJ dysfunction
_____ Multiple trigger points	_____ Myofascial pain syndrome

(Reprinted with permission from Starlanyl and Copeland, 1996)

After you get your healing go back to your Doctor to confirm your healing so he/she can verify that you've been healed. Prove your healing to yourself by using the self-test before and after. If you've had a history of Anxiety Attacks and have finished this program, you need to begin to do things you didn't do before and go where you used to not be able to go before and see for yourself how effective this program has been for you. Each person's healing may vary slightly, but even if you have some residual problems, I'm sure you will agree with what Paul wrote in the Bible in II Corinthians 12:7-9: "And lest I should be exalted above measure through the abundance of the revelations, there was given to me a thorn in the flesh, the messenger of Satan to buffet me, lest I should be exalted above measure. For this thing I besought the Lord thrice, that it might depart from me. And he said unto me, My grace is sufficient for thee: for my strength is made perfect in weakness. Most gladly therefore will I rather glory in my infirmities, that the power of Christ may rest upon me." Paul may have been stuck with a thorn in his flesh but you on the other hand no longer have to stay that way. And if you have any residual problems whatsoever just always remember ". . . my grace is sufficient for thee: for my strength is made perfect in weakness."

CHAPTER 17

Living a Full Life Again

Since I've completed this program, how could I ever tell you about the change that has taken place and about the feeling that goes with that change. It's like metamorphosis of a caterpillar going through the cocoon and blossoming out as a beautiful Black Swallow Tailed butterfly with purple, black and blue colors all blending together across its wings just radiating with awesomeness and beauty. It's like weeping that endured for the night, but then joy came in the morning. One thing is for sure; you'll never know what this truly feels like until you've experienced it for yourself. Trust me. Sometimes there's just no easy way around things. There's just simply no way out except a little hard work. And if we face the music now we'll be joyfully humming the melody in our hearts for the rest of our lives. So I'll see you when you come climbing over the fence where the grass is definitely greener, despite what you've been told. Besides whoever said that the grass wasn't greener on the other side of the fence? Have you ever talked to someone that's been there? I dare these syndromes to ever attack me again with trigger points, tender points or constant pain because I've got a weapon against them now. Currently I don't have a problem worth complaining about. It's like I'm immune to them. Even if they came back, I've got the ultimate weapon to use against them because I now know how to conquer these illnesses.

So why stand halt between two opinions? If you follow through with this program you'll get excellent health benefits that will last the rest of your life. Think about it and weigh it out for yourself: no more tender points, no more trigger points, no more constant widespread musculoskeletal pain, no more anxiety (panic) attacks, and much less fatigue and sleep disturbance. On the other hand, if you don't take action and follow through with this program, you will still be going to doctor after doctor, trying to find relief in medicines that just won't cure Fibromyalgia, Myofascial Pain Syndrome, or any of these other illnesses. So, do you know which option you're going to choose for your life? As for me, there is no choice. I'm going to choose better health at all costs. Besides, the pay off is out of this world. When people get healed, their brain tends to forget all about the pain and suffering they went through. So if you do finish this program remember to take time to reflect on where you used to be and that can help you when you start to plan out where you are going in your future.

We're living in a day and age where information is available at the speed of light across the internet and knowledge is doubling exponentially. To find out all about a subject you can just point and click. But after people have written thousands of books on certain subjects and never seem to come up with a solution is nothing but further evidence of what the Bible says people do in II Tim. 3:7 ". . . ever learning and never able to come to the knowledge of the truth." In Proverbs 4:7 it says "Wisdom is the principal thing; therefore get wisdom: and with all thy getting get understanding." People today think that knowledge is power and load themselves with tons of it. But they seem to lack Godly wisdom which can help them

> *Following through this program is as when a child gets sick and has to take bittersweet cough medicine so he can get well again. He doesn't want to take it, but Dr. Mom knows best and he ends up drinking every last drop. Many days later he's out playing and has forgotten that he was ever even sick.*
>
> R.D.G.

put it all together. Not only do they lack Godly wisdom, but sound judgment and righteous judgment as well. They fail to exercise Godly wisdom to decide how to use their knowledge. In order to exercise knowledge with wisdom you may have to take a step back and use sound judgment in every decision to insure that the best solution is reached and that it will have quality lasting results. Most people can't wait that long so they make quick heady decisions that later may prove to be quite disastrous. Here's the major point, if you want to slow down the driving pace of this world, you're going to have to stop, kneel down and pray. This is your ultimate weapon to use against every problem in the world and yet hardly anybody wants to use it. This is how to get answers from God and not the world through things like the internet. Yes, a lot of the knowledge on the internet can be of some help but without sound Godly wisdom it's only going to create more problems down the road. Those problems will take even longer to fix and then when will people ever have the time to clean up all of the messes that they have made through their poor judgment of decisions?

People with FMS and other illnesses have had things slowed down for them to the point that they just can't afford to make mistakes and would rather have well-thought-out approaches to fixing their short-term problems as well as their long-term problems. This program is a good example of using Godly wisdom and not just worldly knowledge. And so you should use the same idea for planning out the rest of your life.

You've learned how to breathe better, eat better, and even exercise properly for FMS, and these other illnesses. After you've experienced multiple symptomatic relief, I'm sure you'll agree that this program was the greatest tool you've ever used against any of these conditions. So let's all thank God that we have another weapon to fight back against them. A great story of Thankfulness is in Luke 17:11-19, "And it came to pass, as he went to Jerusalem, that he passed through the midst of Samaria and

Galilee. And as he entered into a certain village, there met him ten men that were lepers, which stood afar off: And they lifted up *their* voices, and said, Jesus, Master, have mercy on us. And when he saw *them, he said unto them, Go shew yourselves unto the priests.* And it came to pass, that, as they went, they were cleansed. And one of them, when he saw that he was healed, turned back, and with a loud voice glorified God. And fell down on his face at his feet, giving him thanks: and he was a Samaritan. And Jesus answering said, Were there not ten cleansed? But where *are* the nine? There are not found that returned to give glory to God, save this stranger. And he said unto him, Arise, go thy way: thy faith hath made thee whole."

The main point of the story is that only one out of the ten lepers that were cleansed came back to thank the Lord for making him clean. Furthermore, the Lord made him completely whole unlike the other nine. Let's not forget to thank the lord for having mercy on us all. Now, you can literally throw away all of your crutches, paraphernalia's and whatever else you've been using to help you because you won't need them anymore. And now that you're all better, you might look back and say "Well, I'm glad that's all over with because that sure was some strong medicine," but it's not so bad after all. Especially since you have no more constant pain, or bothersome trigger points or tender points. You're not going to feel as bad as when you had your illness and in addition you're not going to have to perform as much exercise as you did through the training program found in the Remedy. You are now somewhere in between those two points. And stress is easier to deal with. Now you're able to do what you used to do and also do it as much as you used to do it. If you decide to stop the anaerobic exercise after completing this program and your body and health doesn't seem as good as it did, then go back to the proper diet and the breathing exercises. This can make you feel healthier, even if you don't integrate the exercises. The nutrition will be of the highest value and the herbal remedies will help you feel so much better too. This is of good use if you get stressed out for any reason after you've completed the program. So, do what's right to keep living the fullest life possible.

So what things will you be doing in order to be living a full life again?

- going to church
- going to dinners
- helping people
- showing acts of kindness and love
- driving
- going to school
- operate your computer
- go to work
- taking vacations
- raise children

- do household chores
- taking time to smell the roses
- taking time to smell the pizza
- taking time to enjoy a cup of tea
- taking time to give your loved ones gifts
- taking time to give your spouse flowers
- exercising
- sports activities
- pursue hobbies
- entertainment
- amusements
- visit museums
- feel confident about your new strength and wellness
- but being humble enough not to boast because of what you've learned through pain and suffering
- and much more

I urge you to seek God through his word as well because there's so much more to living a beautiful life than just getting physically healed. There's emotional healing, spiritual healing and just getting divinely inspired from time to time, that's a plus and an added benefit all by itself. Take more time to appreciate your better health. Live every minute with enjoyment and make it fulfilling. Don't take your health for granted this time. It's precious.

How much does your health cost? The greatest reward you can have is to regain your life back to the point that you are living a complete and full life again. The greatest reward I can have is knowing that I've helped many others who otherwise were confounded by numerous medical treatments with no real end in sight to regain their health. This creates a win-win situation for everyone.

EPILOGUE

This remedy is not just some cover-up like most medicines but a true remedy for the root of the problem. In Isaiah 59:19 it says, "when the enemy shall come in like a flood, the Spirit of the LORD shall lift up a standard against him (the devil)". FMS (fibromyalgia), MPS (myofascial pain syndrome), CFS (chronic fatigue syndrome), CFIDS (chronic fatigue immuno—dysfunction syndrome), GWS (Gulf War syndrome) and (AA) Anxiety (Panic) Attacks now all have a new standard raised up against them despite their prevalence and annoyance for so long. So I hope you will tell others that they have a fighting chance to prevail against these illnesses. The Bible clearly states that in the last days, knowledge shall increase. It has increased so that you can be helped. I hope this book is your rainbow after the storm. After reading other books on these illnesses, I really didn't get any healthier following their programs (even following religiously). Some people try to impress others with their worldly knowledge and education such as some medical books have done on these very subjects. But the Bible says in I Corinthians 1:19 "For it is written, I will destroy the wisdom of the wise, and will bring to nothing the understanding of the prudent." It also says in I Corinthians 2:4-5, "And my speech and my preaching was not with enticing words of man's wisdom, but in demonstration of the Spirit and of power: that your faith should not stand in the wisdom of men, but in the power of God." Some writers seem to talk all about the subject and yes, you guessed it, they fail to truly find a permanent solution to the problem such as for these conditions. But yet want to be an acclaimed expert on the subject. Then after that, there gets to be too many experts on the same subject and they all have a different variation and there is nothing left over but arguing. Many times there is no solid agreement as to what is absolute. Chaos is about the best way to describe this type of situation.

Many are still hoping that scientists can find the exact etiology of these conditions. I would still love to see a medicine found and prescribed which will act on the neurotransmitters to allow the proper sleep to be restored and to take away the tired feeling that goes along with Fibromyalgia. That would be wonderful, but until then, there's God's Remedy. There is probably billions of dollars being spent on research at this time and none of the big money researchers have discovered God's Remedy. It didn't take a lot of gold or silver to learn this because it came from God. James 1:17 says that "every good and perfect gift . . . cometh from above, from the father of lights . . ." and *a gift is free!*

> The answer to every problem you'll ever encounter is already written in the Holy Bible.
>
> *R.D.G.*

It's not enough just to survive FMS, MPS, CFS, etc. We Christians need to have enough power through God to be more than a conqueror over illnesses, diseases and all types of infirmities. And even if God doesn't heal you or me of anything else, He is still a healer.

The hours you put into this program are almost nothing compared to how good you will feel the rest of your life once you become more than a conqueror too. Jesus Christ can heal any and all sicknesses and diseases.

I believe the apostle James summed it up best in James 2:18 when he said, ". . . Shew me thy faith without thy works, and I will shew thee my faith by my works . . . ," because "faith without works is dead, being alone" (James 2:17). If you've got the faith to believe for something, He's got the power to bring it to pass. I've got medical records dating back to January 1997 that show that I in fact checked out with no more tender points and no more trigger points. I originally finished this program in 1996, and still have no sign of trigger points or tender points today. I seem to have forgotten that I once had these conditions. Now I know God healed me and I have proof that virtually all signs and symptoms aren't there (except for small residual inconveniences). So try God's Remedy. You'll be amazed at the results. No more constant musculoskeletal pain, no more tender points, no more trigger points and no more Anxiety (Panic) Attacks.

> When telling someone how to be healed you can't just focus on one aspect such as the physical symptoms. One must take the person as a whole into consideration and deal with the spirit, soul, mind and body in order to achieve a total sense of well being.
>
> R.D.G.

Everything is there, the protein drinks, the supplements, the exercise regimen and the hot tub therapy. I've made it easy, all you have to do is follow the exercises and go through the entire program.

I just told you what God did for me in my life and what he is able to do for you in your life. My prayer is that you get your miracle but like the Lord warned don't tell anyone else about your healing or the name of that Great Physician, Jesus Christ, because they probably won't believe you anyway. People can be very skeptical. But I do pray that you enjoy your newfound health. The only part I feel sad about is that everyone may not be able to perform this program from start to finish and probably due to some other type of injury or illness. Not only do I try to motivate people to deal with their physical illness, but to deal with their mind, soul and spirit to encourage them that God does have a Remedy for these illnesses and it was only a matter of time and prayer before someone discovered it. For it says in James 1:5 "If any of you lack wisdom, let him ask of God, that giveth to all men liberally, and upbraideth not; and it shall be given him." Then in Jeremiah 33:3, "Call unto me and I will answer thee and show thee great and mighty things, which thou knowest not."

So with this book I would like to leave patients with encouragement and hope. I truly felt obligated to share this book with not only all of the patients, but the whole world. Keep in mind that the cost of this book is less than the cost of an office visit with your physician. It's truly been a privilege and an honor to teach and share what God has revealed to me. May God Bless You.

The End.

Update: Since the writing of this book, it was revealed to me that the disability and psychiatric symptoms I had starting in 1988 were related to taking dangerous diet pills. I had taken Extra Strength Dexatrim diet pills which contained Phenylpropanolamine (PPA) and in November, 2000 the FDA requested all pharmaceutical companies to voluntarily withdraw the marketing of this drug due to its tendency to cause hemorrhagic strokes, psychosis and even death. This was also the cause of that mysterious 4 year constant headache that I had suffered with. An MRI had revealed two possible microvascular events in the brain.

So not only did I have damage from PPA, but I also had FMS, MPS, CFS and AA on top of it all.

Despite all of that, I kept only just believing and eventually discovered this Remedy which is helping so many people today.

Appendix A

Part 1 Suppliers of Health Care Products for the Consumer

I. Products

AMERICAN SPORTS NUTRITION, INC.
1501 East Main St.
Meriden, CT 06450 USA
(makers of American Whey™)
Phone: 1(888) 462-5671
International: 1(203) 639-8189
Fax: 1(203) 639-8089
Email: *american.sports@americanwhey.com*
    customerservice@americanwhey.com
    sales@americanwhey.com

COUNTRY LIFE VITAMINS
101 Corporate Drive
Hauppauge, NY 11788
(*makers of vitamins and nutritional supplements*)
Toll Free: 1(800) 645-5768
International: 1(631) 231-1031
http://www.country-life.com

VNF NUTRITION
246 RT 25 A
East Setauket, NY 11733
Toll Free: 1(800) 681-7099
International: 1(631) 689-6433
Mon.-Fri. 9:00 a.m. to 5:00 p.m. EST
Fax: 1(631) 689-7638
Email: *VNF@village.com*
http://www.VNFNUTRITION.com
(*suppliers of Nutritional products*)

Appendix B

GOD'S REMEDY

Name _____ Date _____ Weight _____

Take all around multi-vitamin, COQ10, Ginkgo Biloba, ½ protein drink— 1 hr. before workout Warm-up 10-15 minutes—aerobic exercise	Dumbbell Weight	Barbell Weight	Machine Weight
Squat			
Leg curl			
Leg curl variation			
Bench press			
Overhead barbell press			
Upright row			
Shrugs			
Barbell row			
Lat pull down			
Hyperextension/Low back machine			
Triceps extension			
Barbell curl			
Reverse curl			
Wrist curl/Reverse wrist curl			
Handgrip exercise			
Calf raise/Toe press			
Shin exercise			
Toe crunch/Toe spread			
Machine crunch/Cross crunch			
Alternate leg kick			
Side bends			

Neck exercises (all 4)			
Eye exercise			
Pucker exercise			
Opening jaw exercise			
Closing jaw exercise			
Fish hook exercise			
Frontalis exercise			
Occipitalis exercise			
Temporalis exercise			
Advanced sprint			
(only occasionally and on Aerobic workout days only)			
Warm down 10 – 15 minutes			
Sauna bath 10 minutes then Cool Down			
Hot tub 10 minutes then shower			
Take 1 protein drink w/meal after workout			
Take 1 protein drink 1 hr. before bedtime			
Rest Plenty			

APPENDIX C

Kit #1

4 month complete supply kit

133 day 25lbs. American Whey™ (about 3 per day)

2 x 60 day supply of C_0Q_{10} 100mg. Country Life® (1 per day)

2 x 60 day supply of Ginkgo Biloba Country Life® (1 per day)

2 x 60 day supply of Daily Total One Rapid Release with or without Iron all around multiple vitamin Country Life® (1 per day)

Kit #2

4 month maintenance kit

160 day 10lbs. Bucket of American Whey™ (about 1 per day)

2 x 60 day supply of C0Q10 100mg. Country Life® (1 per day)

2 x 60 day supply of Daily Total One Rapid Release with or without Iron all around multiple vitamin Country Life® (1 per day)

BIBLIOGRAPHY

All scripture quotations are taken from the Holy Bible, King James Version.

"Alexander Fleming." *Hutchinson Dictionary of Scientific Biography.* The McGaw-Hill companies. 10 April 2000. On-line 08 February 2002. http://www.accessscience.com/server-java/Arknoid/science/AS/ Biographies/3/231.html

American College of Rheumatology, Arthritis & Rheumatism, 1990: 33(2); 160-172, FG-1 with permission from Lippincott, Willims & Wilkins (LWW)

American Psychiatric Association: Diagnostic and Statistical Manual of Mental Disorders (DSM-IV). Ed 4. Washington, DC, American Psychiatric Association, 1994, pp. 393-405.

Arthritis Foundation®, *Fibromyalgia Syndrome*, Atlanta, GA. Arthritis Foundation, 1998, pp.2-3+

Berkow, Robert ed. Fletcher, Andrew J. ed. *Fifteenth edition, The Merck Manual of Diagnosis and Therapy*, Rahway, N.J. Merck and Co., Inc. 1987

CFIDS Research. *Google.* 2001. *CFIDS Association of America.* On-line, 13 June 2001. *http://cfids.org*

"Charles Goodyear." *Improvements in India-Rubber Fabrics.*" National Inventors Hall of Fame. Akron, OH, U.S. Patent and trademark office, U.S.A., 02 November 2001. On-line 04 February 2002. *http://www.invent.org/book/book-text/47html*

Clarke J N. The search for Legitimacy and the "expertization" of the layperson: the case of chronic fatigue syndrome. *Social work in health care.* 2000; vol. 30, no. 3, 73-93

Consensus Document on Fibromyalgia: The Copenhagen Declaration. Issued by the Second World Congress on Myofascial Pain and Fibromyalgia meeting August 17-20,

1992. Published *Lancet,* vol. 340, Sept. 12, 1992, and incorporated into the World Health Organization's 10th revision of the International Statistical Classification of Diseases and Related Health Problems, ICD 10, Jan. 1, 1993. Available from Bente Dannesdiold-Samsøe, Department of Rheumatology, Frederiksberg Hospital, Ndr Fasanvej 57, DK-2000 Frederiksberg, Denmark. Also in the *Journal of Musculoskeletal Pain,* vol. 1, No. 3 / 4, 1993.

Davidson, Paul, Chronic Muscle Pain Syndrome. New York: Villard Books, 1989, p. 25

Eichner, Edward R., "Use fitness to fight fibromyalgia." *YOUR PATIENT & FITNESS* Vol. 4, No. 6. November 1990: pp. 19+

Fomby, Elizabeth W., Mellion, Morris B., "Identifying and Treating Myofascial Pain Syndrome." *THE PHYSICIAN AND SPORTS MEDICINE.* Feb. 1997: Vol. 25, No. 2, Google.com on-line. 07 Jan. 2001 [http://www.physsportsmed.com]

Foods that Harm, Foods that Heal. Pleasantville, NY, Readers Digest, 1997

"Frequently Asked Questions." *Gulf Vets.* 24 May 2001. 10 July 2001. *http://www.va.gov/heatlh/environ/persgulf.htm*

Fulcher KY, White PD. Strength and physiological response to exercise in patients with chronic fatigue syndrome. (Journal of Neurology, Neurosurgery and Psychiatry 2000; 69:302-7)

"Gulf War Syndrome." *The Biofact Report.* On-line 12 July 2001. *http://www.biofact.com/*

Hendrix ML. Understanding Panic Disorder. National Institute of Mental Health. NIH Publication. No. 93-3509. 1993.

Hunt SC. "The Gulf War Syndrome controversy." *School of Hygiene and Public Health of the Johns Hopkins University.* 1999. Vol. 150. No. 2. pp. 216-217.

Kaires P. "Symptons in Persian Gulf War Veterans." *Journal of Occupational and environmental medicine.* 1999. Vol. 41. No. 11. pp. 939

Kennedy, Robert and Greenwood-Robinson, Maggie, *Built! The new body building for everyone,* New York, Perigee Books, 1987

Krsnich-Shriwise, Susan. "Fibromyalgia syndrome: an overview." *American Physical Therapy Associates,* (Vol. 77, No. 1 Jan. 1997)

Lane R., Chronic Fatigue syndrome: is it physical? Journal of Neurology, Neurosurgery and Psychiatry 2000; 69:289

Lee, William., Coenzyme Q-10, Is it our new fountain of youth? New Canaan, CT, Keats Publishing Inc., 1987

"Managing your Fatigue." *Arthritis Foundation.* 1997.

McCauley LA, Joos Sk, Lasarev MR, Storzbach D, Bourdette DN. "Gulf war unexplained illnesses: persistence and unexplained nature of self-reported symptoms." *Environmental research.* 1999. Vol. 81. No. 3. pp. 215-223

Merritt TC. "Recognition and acute management of patients with panic attacks in emergency department." *Emergency medical clinics of North America.* 2000. Vol. 18. No. 2. pp. 289-300.

Ohayon MM, Shapiro CM. Sleep and Fatigue. Seminars in Clinical Neuropsychiatry. 2000; Vol. 5, No. 1, 56-57

"Operation Mission Impossible." *Gulf war veteran Resource pages.* 1994-2001. Google. com. 23 July 2001. *http://www.gulfweb.org/*

Paluska SA, Schwenk TL. "Physical activity and mental health current concepts." *Sports Medicine.* 2000. Vol. 29. Issue 3. pp. 167-180

"Researchers Find Abnormality in Fibromyalgia," American College of Rheumatology, 26 April 2001. on-line 11 March 2002 [http://rheumatology.org/press/nm96/fibrox.htm

Rosenberg RN, Paty DW. "Defining the neurological basis of the Gulf War Syndrome." *Archives of Neurology.* 2000. Vol. 57. No. 9. pp. 1263.

Starlaynl, Devin and Copeland, Mary Ellen, *Fibromyalgia & Chronic Myofascial Pain Syndrome; A Survivor's Manual.* New Harbinger Publications, Inc. 1996.

"The Physiology of Hot water." What happens to your body when you soak in Hot water. Pool & Spa News. On-line 8 January 2001. http://www.ybtubless.com/hotwater.htm

Tierney, Lawrence M., Jr., McPhee, Stephen J., Papadakis, Maxine A., *Current Medical Diagnosis and treatment,* Stamford, CT: Appleton and Large, A Simon and Schuster Co., 1998, p. 788

Travell, Janet G. and David G. Simons. Myofascial Pain and Dysfunction: The Trigger Point Manual. Volume I; The Upper Body, Baltimore, MD: Williams and Wilkins, 1983.

Travell, Janet G. and David G. Simons, Myofascial Pain and Dysfunction: The Trigger Point Manual. Volume II: The Lower Body. Baltimore, MD: Williams and Wilkins, 1992

"UT Southwestern team traces Gulf War illnesses to chemicals: Three primary syndromes identified." *Southwestern.* 14 Feb. 1997. On-line 13 July 2001. http://www.swmed.edu/home_pages

VGM's Careers Encyclopedia. Lincolnwood (Chicago, IL): NTC Publishing Group. 1997

Williamson, Miryam E., *Fibromyalgia, a comprehensive approach.* New York, NY, Markham, ON., Walker and Company, Thomas Allen and Son, Canada, 1996

World Book Encyclopedia, Chicago, U.S.A. Field Enterprises, 1977, N-O, Q-R.

Advertisement for purchase of other Books

"The Lord Loveth a cheerful giver"

If you've had success and have recovered from any of these illnesses then mail me a postcard stating so.

If you've benefited or have been blessed in any way from this book and you would like to sow a special love gift offering, please send it to:

Rod Gatti Ministries
c/o Xlibris Corporation
1663 Liberty Drive
Bloomington, IN 47403

I'm enclosing my check or money order for: ⌐ $25.00   ⌐ $50.00
⌐ $100.00   ⌐ other $_____

"Give and it shall be given . . ."